Breastfeeding Challenges Made Easy
for Late Preterm Infants

Sandra Cole, RNC, IBCLC, began her career as a neonatal intensive care nurse at the Royal Alexandra Hospital in Edmonton, Alberta, Canada, in 1990. In 1992, she moved to the United States where she continued in neonatal nursing until 2010, working at the University Medical Center in Lubbock, Texas, Chester County Hospital in West Chester, Pennsylvania, Pascack Valley Hospital in Westwood, New Jersey, and Good Samaritan Hospital in Suffern, New York. She held many positions such as staff nurse, preceptor, charge nurse, transport nurse, and extracorporeal membrane oxygenation (ECMO) technician and earned the Neonatal Intensive Care Nursing Certification in 2003.

Despite the myriad obstacles sick babies face while in the neonatal intensive care unit (NICU), one of the most frustrating situations for Ms. Cole to witness was late preterm infants struggling with breastfeeding. Realizing that these babies required specialized breastfeeding assistance, she chose to pursue the path of lactation consultant in order to better understand the breastfeeding needs of these babies and to become better equipped to assist in the transition to exclusive breastfeeding in this population. In 2007, Ms. Cole earned her international board-certified lactation consultant (IBCLC) certificate and started a successful private lactation practice in New York where she specialized in late preterm infants. It was through working with these late preterm infants that her strategies for successful breastfeeding were developed and fine tuned.

Ms. Cole is currently working as part of the lactation team at Sharp Mary Birch Hospital where she continues to advance her knowledge base and inspire breastfeeding parents.

Breastfeeding Challenges Made Easy for Late Preterm Infants

The Go-To Guide for Nurses and Lactation Consultants

Sandra Cole, RNC, IBCLC

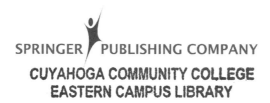

SPRINGER PUBLISHING COMPANY

Springer Publishing Company, LLC
11 West 42nd Street
New York, NY 10036
www.springerpub.com

Acquisitions Editor: Elizabeth Nieginski
Composition: Graphic World

ISBN: 978-0-8261-9603-3
e-book ISBN: 978-0-8261-9604-0

13 14 15 / 5 4 3 2 1

The author and the publisher of this Work have made every effort to use sources believed to be reliable to provide information that is accurate and compatible with the standards generally accepted at the time of publication. The author and publisher shall not be liable for any special, consequential, or exemplary damages resulting, in whole or in part, from the readers' use of, or reliance on, the information contained in this book. The publisher has no responsibility for the persistence or accuracy of URLs for external or third-party Internet websites referred to in this publication and does not guarantee that any content on such websites is, or will remain, accurate or appropriate.

Library of Congress Cataloging-in-Publication Data

Cole, Sandra, 1967- author.
  Breastfeeding challenges made easy for late preterm infants : the go-to guide for nurses and lactation consultants / Sandra Cole.
    p. ; cm.
  Includes bibliographical references and index.
  ISBN 978-0-8261-9603-3 — ISBN 978-0-8261-9604-0 (e-book)
  I. Title.
  [DNLM: 1. Breast Feeding—methods. 2. Infant Care—methods. 3. Infant, Premature—physiology. 4. Maternal-Child Nursing—standards. WS 125]
  RJ216
  613.2'69—dc23
                          2013037343

Special discounts on bulk quantities of our books are available to corporations, professional associations, pharmaceutical companies, health care organizations, and other qualifying groups. If you are interested in a custom book, including chapters from more than one of our titles, we can provide that service as well.

For details, please contact:
Special Sales Department, Springer Publishing Company, LLC
11 West 42nd Street, 15th Floor, New York, NY 10036-8002
Phone: 877-687-7476 or 212-431-4370; Fax: 212-941-7842
E-mail: sales@springerpub.com

Printed in the United States of America by Edwards Brothers Malloy.

To all the late preterm infants and their families whom I have had the pleasure to work with throughout the years, thank you for enlightening me.

Contents

Foreword Barbara Morrison, PhD, APRN-CNM   *ix*
Preface   *xiii*
Acknowledgments   *xvii*

Part I: Physiological Challenges That Undermine Successful
     Breastfeeding for the Late Preterm Infant
Prologue

Special Characteristics of the Late Preterm Infant

Chapter 1: Defining the Late Preterm Infant   *3*

Chapter 2: Risk Factors for Late Preterm Births   *9*

Specific Physiological Challenges for the Late Preterm Infant

Chapter 3: Immature Neurological Development and Hypotonia   *17*

Chapter 4: Temperature Instability, Hypoglycemia, and Increased
     Metabolism   *25*

Chapter 5: Hyperbilirubinemia   *33*

Chapter 6: Unstable Respiratory Status   *41*

Chapter 7: Increased Risk for Infection   *49*

Maternal Conditions Affecting Breastfeeding Success

Chapter 8: Maternal Conditions Affecting Breast Milk Supply   *53*

Chapter 9: Maternal Self-Esteem and Its Effect on Breastfeeding   *65*

Chapter 10: The Risks of Not Breastfeeding   *69*

Part II: Conquering Breastfeeding Challenges for the Late Preterm Infant
Prologue

Setting the Stage for Successfully Breastfeeding the Late Preterm Infant

Chapter 11: Health Initiatives   *81*

Chapter 12: Early and Frequent Breastfeeding   *89*

Specific Strategies for Overcoming Breastfeeding Challenges

Chapter 13: Decrease Stimuli and Energy Expenditure   *95*

Chapter 14: Proper Positioning and Latch Technique   *103*

Chapter 15: Breast Compressions   *115*

Chapter 16: Nipple Shields   *121*

Chapter 17: Breast Pumps   *137*

Chapter 18: Breast Massage and Hand Expression   *153*

Chapter 19: Supplemental Feedings   *161*

Encouragement for a Successful Breastfeeding Experience

Chapter 20: Overcoming Other Challenges   *175*

Chapter 21: Maternal Satisfaction and Breastfeeding Success: The Big Picture   *181*

Chapter 22: Putting It All Together: Summary of Important Highlights for Successful Breastfeeding for Late Preterm Infants   *185*

Appendix A: Late Preterm Infant Breastfeeding Algorithm   191
Appendix B: Sample In-Hospital Late Preterm Infant Initiative   193
Appendix C: Follow-Up Care of the Breastfeeding Late Preterm Infant   199
Appendix D: Sample Patient Teaching Handout: Your Late Preterm Infant   201
Appendix E: Sample Late Preterm Infant Feeding Plan   203

References   205

Additional Reading   227

Resources for Nurses and Parents   235

Index   239

Foreword

Breastfeeding is one of the greatest gifts a mother can give to her newborn baby. Breastfeeding and skin-to-skin holding, or kangaroo care, provide ongoing nutrition and nurturance, enhancing cardiorespiratory and metabolic stability during the immediate postpartum period (birth through the first few days of life) and increasing maturation of immature body systems as newborns continue to adapt to life outside the womb (American Academy of Pediatrics, 2012). In their natural habitat, with kangaroo care, newborn infants are maintained in a neutral thermal environment; they have ready access to food and move to the breast with minimal assistance; gain protection from acute infections and many chronic illnesses through colostrum, breast milk, and skin-to-skin contact; and hear sounds and smell odors that are familiar because of experiences in the womb. Additionally, bonding, social and emotional regulation, and cognitive and language development are facilitated through maternal–infant interactions spontaneously occurring in kangaroo care. However, infants born early, between 34 0/7 and 36 6/7 weeks gestation and known as late preterm infants (LPIs; Phillips, 2013), and their mothers have unique challenges when trying to adapt to extra-uterine life. While LPIs look like full-term newborns (37 0/7 to 41 6/7 weeks gestation), they are physiologically and metabolically less mature, frequently with insufficient self-regulatory abilities to react to the demands of life outside the uterus (Phillips, 2013). Due to their immaturity, breastfeeding challenges are common for mother–LPI dyads but may go unrecognized, secondary to health care providers' lack of awareness and identification of potential risks for LPIs and timely intervention.

Breastfeeding Challenges Made Easy for Late Preterm Infants is an important, evidence-based primer for nurses, midwives, nurse practitioners, physician assistants, lactation consultants, physicians, and other health care providers supporting and encouraging breastfeeding efforts of mother–LPI dyads. Sandra Cole brings her expertise as a lactation consultant, with many years of practical, hands-on clinical experience, to the creation of this book. Cole has incorporated the newly revised *Multidisciplinary Guidelines for Care of Late Preterm Infants* from the National Perinatal Association (Phillips et al., 2013), which reiterates the tenets of the Baby-Friendly Hospital Initiative (World Health Organization [WHO], UNICEF, & Wellstart, 2009) and the Mother-Friendly Childbirth Initiative (Coalition for Improving Maternity Services [CIMS], 1996). All three documents define optimal care for mother–infant dyads through birth and postpartum, and strongly recommend 24-hour rooming-in with frequent, prolonged kangaroo care to promote optimal physiological stability and to facilitate breastfeeding. Cole elaborates on the aforementioned guidelines by elucidating the physiological and developmental challenges of LPIs that could undermine breastfeeding initiation and success. In Part II of the book, Cole provides evidence-based suggestions for overcoming the challenges.

Birthing their babies before the estimated due date, even if it is just by a few weeks, is a crisis for mothers and their significant others. One way mothers can allay the guilt and grave concerns regarding the health of their newborns is by being actively involved in their infants' care. Only mothers can provide the optimal habitat with kangaroo care and breastfeeding. But health care providers can optimize the dyadic experience by promptly identifying physiological, developmental, and lactation challenges and finding ways to overcome the challenges so mother and infant can stay together. *Breastfeeding Challenges Made Easy for Late Preterm Infants* is a resource presented in a timely way so the most up-to-date, evidence-based care is provided to LPIs in the hospital and after discharge. And perhaps the guidance and suggestions provided by Cole for LPIs can also improve breastfeeding care and provide support to full-term mother–infant dyads as well as mother–preterm infant dyads.

Barbara Morrison, PhD, APRN-CNM
Associate Professor
Janice M. Riordan Distinguished Professorship
Wichita State University, School of Nursing
Wichita, Kansas

REFERENCES

American Academy of Pediatrics, Section on Breastfeeding. (2012). Breastfeeding and the use of human milk. *Pediatrics, 129,* e827. doi: 10.1542/peds.2011-3552

Coalition for Improving Maternity Services. (1996). *Mother-Friendly Childbirth Initiative.* Retrieved from http://www.motherfriendly.org/MFCI

Phillips, R. M. (2013). Introduction, Multidisciplanary guidelines for the care of late preterm infants. *Journal of Perinatology 33,* S3–S4. doi:10.1038/jp.2013.52

Phillips, R.M., Goldstein, M., Hougland, K., Nandyal, R., Pizzica, A., Santa-Donato, A., Staebler, S., Stark, A.R., Treiger, T.M., & Yost, E. on behalf of The National Perinatal Association. (2013). Practice guidelines: Multidisciplinary guidelines for the care of late preterm infants. *Journal of Perinatology 33,* S5–S22. doi:10.1038/jp.2013.53

World Health Organization (WHO), UNICEF, & Wellstart International. (2009). Baby-Friendly Hospital Initiative (BFHI): Revised, updated and expanded for integrated care. Section 1: Background and implementation. Geneva, Switzerland: WHO Press.

Preface

In 2010, while working as a nurse in the neonatal intensive care unit (NICU) of Good Samaritan Hospital in Suffern, New York, I was asked by Anne Jorgensen, a neonatal nurse practitioner, to present a 10-minute slide presentation to the staff outlining the difficulties late preterm infants have with breastfeeding and the strategies needed to overcome these difficulties. While putting the slides together, I realized there was no way the presentation would take only 10 minutes. The outline of the problems these babies face would take at least that long to present and the strategies to overcome these breastfeeding challenges would take a minimum of another 20 minutes without going into any details. At that point I knew I had the beginnings of a journal article, and began filling in the outline, planning to write my first journal article.

The reality hit me soon after. There was much too much information to cover, even if I wrote a series of journal articles.

So the outline continued to evolve into chapters, and the chapters continued to develop into a book manuscript.

At that time, late preterm infants were automatically admitted to the NICU, where they were cared for until they proved themselves to be capable of breastfeeding effectively, or at least able to take full feedings by bottle, then discharged directly to home. The struggle to get these babies to breastfeed was witnessed firsthand by those working in the NICU and by the parents of these babies. Discharge follow-up was often done with the neonatologist or neonatal clinic specializing in caring for late preterm infants, and not with general pediatricians, as is common today.

Soon after, things changed. Medical advances in prenatal care decreased the severity of respiratory and other complications in late preterm infants in the immediate period after birth. As a result, medical insurers, obstetricians, pediatricians, postpartum nurses, and parents often viewed late preterm infants as just smaller versions of term babies. Late preterm infants were often cared for on the general postpartum unit, discharged home at the same time as the mother, and discharge follow-up was done at the pediatrician's office. These babies were only admitted to the NICU if they were in respiratory distress or if they continued to exhibit abnormal glucose control, temperature instability, or signs of sepsis. Hyperbilirubinemia was often treated at home with bili-blankets— and so the challenges began to be seen.

During that time period, some misconceptions about late preterm infants began to arise. It was assumed that sleepy babies would wake up when they were hungry enough, babies who were not vigorous at the breast were called "lazy," and mothers were often made to feel inadequate for not having a full milk supply or not feeding their babies often enough. At the same time, babies were losing weight and facing many serious complications. The incidence of hospital readmissions for late preterm infants began to rapidly increase, and many mothers were forced to give up breastfeeding in order to accurately measure nutritional intake, to supply their baby with enough calories for proper growth, and to decrease the severity of complications. Caring for late preterm infants became an uphill struggle for the babies, the families, the nursing staff, and the pediatricians.

The emotional frustration, financial toll, and long-term outcomes associated with late preterm infants are now among the hot topics at conferences, in journal articles, and among pediatricians and medical insurance companies. Most medical professionals recognize the challenges late preterm infants face, and recognize that most of these challenges can be minimized by early, effective breastfeeding. However, until this book, very little information was available as to *how* to achieve effective breastfeeding in this population.

This book's foundation is supported by evidence-based research, and backed by decades of working with late preterm infants in the NICU, the regular nursery and postpartum units, as well as in the home setting, long term, after discharge from the hospital.

My hope is that *Breastfeeding Challenges Made Easy for Late Preterm Infants* gives all those caring for late preterm infants and their families the knowledge needed to understand why and how these babies differ from full-term breastfeeding infants, as well as a thorough understanding of the strategic techniques required for overcoming these challenges.

While this book was written specifically for breastfeeding late preterm infants, the techniques to successful breastfeeding described in this book can be used for any baby who is having challenges with effective breastfeeding. As we know, change is constant. There are ongoing opportunities for evidence-based research to guide us to provide the best care to all our patients.

Sandra Cole

Acknowledgments

I am indebted to my editor, Elizabeth Nieginski, at Springer Publishing Company for recognizing the timely importance of this book.

I would also like to thank my husband and my children for putting up with my obsession to finish writing this book. They have been well educated on the importance of effective breastfeeding, and my son has been exposed to more breastfeeding information than any teenage boy would care to know. My daughter has been my sounding board and was instrumental in obtaining the perfect photographs of breastfeeding equipment. My husband tirelessly helped me through computer glitches.

PART I Physiological Challenges That Undermine Successful Breastfeeding for the Late Preterm Infant

Prologue

Doctors and neonatal nurses have only recently recognized the challenges that late preterm infants face when transitioning to extra-uterine life. The medical community is becoming aware that these babies exhibit health complications that differ in timing, severity, and outcomes from preterm babies, and even though late preterm infants might initially appear to be smaller full-term babies, the greatest amount of health care spending on newborns is on these babies who are born at 34 to 36 6/7 weeks gestation. With hospital discharges occurring within 24 to 72 hours after birth, the complications related to late preterm births often go unrecognized by hospital staff, assuming erroneously that these babies will fare well once home.

Thirteen percent of these late preterm infants are readmitted to hospitals within the first few weeks after discharge because of serious complications caused by disturbances of respiratory, metabolic, neurological, and immunological function specific to being born at late preterm gestation. Most of these disturbances can be exaggerated by poor breastfeeding, also specific to this population of infants.

Late preterm infants face myriad complications, but if they are not displaying visible complications such as respiratory distress, health care professionals often overlook the seriousness of the less visible complications such as hypoglycemia, infection, temperature instability, dehydration, and jaundice that signal a decreased ability to react and adapt to extra-uterine life and are common to late preterm infants. If immediate action to overcome the cascade of metabolic, neurological, and immunological disturbances is not taken, late preterm infants are placed at a great disadvantage, affecting not just short-term outcomes but long-term sequelae as well. Short-term consequences include rehospitalization for intravenous antibiotics, phototherapy, or intravenous hydration. Long-term consequences include failure to thrive, impairments of normal childhood development, cardiac or respiratory failure, mental retardation, cerebral palsy, and possible death.

There are many causes for the increased incidence of late preterm births, including increased use and development of medical technologies for pregnancy and labor. Late preterm births are on the rise in many countries, and in 2009, 9% of all births in the United States were late preterm infants.

Anne Jorgenson (2008) once stated that this group of vulnerable infants follow the four U's: underestimated, understudied, unpredictable, and unrecognized. Although that was true at the time of her research, the medical community has now come to realize that late preterm infants are *overestimated* in their abilities to effectively breastfeed and maintain extra-uterine homeostasis, are *predictable* in their outcomes of breastfeeding complications and morbidities and timing of these complications, and are fully *recognized* in such a way that we now know that each of these babies face an uphill battle with disturbances in normal fetal-to-newborn adaptation, requiring breastfeeding assistance geared specifically to each individual baby and his or her ability to breastfeed at any given feeding time. It is the medical professionals who are caring for these babies who are unpredictable in terms of their approach to care, unrecognizing of the assistance required for these breastfeeding babies, and who underestimate the seriousness of ineffective breastfeeding in the late preterm population and how they can assist these babies to overcome the difficulties associated with breastfeeding.

With this book, hopefully those hundreds of thousands of late preterm infants born every year and their parents will be better prepared for the realities of the transition from in utero to extra-uterine life. Nurses and lactation consultants, as well as physicians and other auxiliary medical personnel, should gain a better understanding of the nuances of this special group of babies. Breastfeeding is one of the most important aspects to late preterm infant care, for both immediate and long-term health outcomes, and with the right approach, it can be done effectively and successfully without complications generally associated with late preterm infants.

ONE

Defining the Late Preterm Infant

WHO IS THE LATE PRETERM INFANT?

Late preterm infants have come under scrutiny over the past few years because of their complicated and often ill-treated course of adaptation to extra-uterine life. They have caused much discussion and research, large health care expenditures, and stress to their families and health care providers because of their high risk of morbidities and mortality.

Late preterm infants are born between 34 0/7 and 36 6/7 weeks gestation, which is 3 to 6 weeks before their intended incubation period of 40 weeks in utero. As a result of their early arrival, requisite maturation of many systems is interrupted, and therefore adaptation to normal processes required for extra-uterine life is hindered. Assuming normal adaptation to life and providing minimal intervention has been the usual course of treatment, especially if the late preterm infant is breathing without difficulty at birth, but this assumption has proven to be harmful to the late preterm population. The medical community has come to realize that late preterm infants are not just smaller versions of full-term infants, and they do not follow the same path of complications that younger preterm infants experience. Late preterm infants require their own set of standards, monitoring, expectations, and outcomes.

A NEW DEFINITION TO CLEARLY DEFINE THE CHALLENGES

Once referred to as "early term" or "near term" infants, late preterm infants were treated as small full-term babies who needed just a little more monitoring in terms of temperature stability, respiratory efforts, and bilirubin clearance. In 2005 the National Institute of Child Health and Human Development assembled a multidisciplinary team of experts for a workshop to improve the care and outcome of these infants. Their goal was to address the issues associated with late preterm infants not normally linked to term infants, such as higher frequency of respiratory distress, apnea, temperature instability, hypoglycemia, seizures, jaundice and kernicterus, feeding problems, and higher rates of rehospitalization (Raju, Higgins, Stark, & Leveno, 2006). Dropping the previous nomenclature, which was misleading, the panel of experts adopted the designation *late preterm*, emphasizing the negative results of underestimation of risks and encouraging more diligent care in terms of evaluation, monitoring, and follow-up. The designation *late preterm* is also ideal because these babies often exhibit complications similar to preterm infants but at a later time frame, often after discharge from the hospital.

INCIDENCE OF LATE PRETERM DELIVERIES

As noted in a National Center for Health Statistics (NCHS) data brief (Martin, Kirmeyer, Osterman, & Shepherd, 2009), trends in birth rates in the United States show that late preterm births rose 20% from 1990 to 2006. On average, there are more than 900 late preterm births per day, or roughly one third of a million (333,461) late preterm births per year in the United States alone. This number is staggering because late preterm infants are more likely than term infants to have complications at birth, require longer and more intensive hospitalization, incur higher medical costs, and have more devastating long-term sequelae. According to the same data brief (Martin et al., 2009), mothers younger than age 20 or older than 40 years are most likely to have a late preterm baby. In addition, in 2006 non-Hispanic Black mothers were about 50% more likely than non-Hispanic White mothers and one third more likely than Hispanic mothers to deliver a late preterm infant.

Thankfully, the rising trend of late preterm births has begun to decline in the United States since 2006 (Martin, Osterman, & Sutton, 2010), possibly as a result of increased awareness of the mortality and morbidity risks that these babies face, and the delay of elective cesarean sections and labor inductions until the baby is further along in development. Late preterm deliveries in 2008 were down 3% from 2006 (Martin et al., 2010) and continued to decline in 2009 (Martin et al., 2011).

WORLDWIDE STATISTICS FOR LATE PRETERM BIRTHS

Late preterm births are not just an issue in the United States but are an epidemic worldwide. In a study published in *The Lancet* (Blencowe et al., 2012), moderate or late preterm births (grouped in a category from 32 to less than 37 weeks) constituted 84% of all preterm births encountered in the 41 countries surveyed during 2010. The study further indicated that the chance of survival for a baby born at 34 weeks in low-income and middle-income countries was only 50%, the equivalent of a 24-week-gestation baby's chance of survival in most high-income countries. The areas with the greatest number of late preterm births (again, categorized as 32 weeks to less than 37 weeks, not 34 weeks to less than 37 weeks as this group is defined in the United States) were Southern Asia, followed by sub-Saharan Africa, Southeastern Asia and Oceania, Central and Eastern Asia, Latin America and the Caribbean and, finally, Northern Africa and Western Asia.

The World Health Organization (WHO, 2012) lists the countries with the greatest number of moderate to late preterm births (32 to less than 37 weeks, not 34 to less than 37 weeks) annually as India with 2,959,300; followed by China with 981,050; Nigeria, 665,080; Pakistan, 633,640; Indonesia, 564,350; United States, 438,410; Bangladesh, 355,030; the Philippines, 295,780; Democratic Republic of the Congo, 291,750; and Brazil, 233,320.

Significance of the Statistics

The reason these statistics are so astonishing and concerning is that late preterm infants face a much greater risk of morbidities and mortality than their full-term counterparts, causing increased stress to the family, increased burdens on the health care system, and even increased demand on society as we begin to see the economic and emotional costs of complications from morbidities when these infants progress from infancy through school-age years and beyond.

Shapiro-Mendoza et al. (2008) determined that morbidity rates during birth hospitalization of term infants born between 38 and 40 weeks gestation was approximately 3%, but then approximately doubled for each additional gestational week earlier than 38 weeks. At 37 weeks they reported a 5.9% morbidity rate and a whopping 51.7%

at 34 weeks. Infants born at 34 weeks had 20 times the risk of morbidities compared to those born at 40 weeks; those born at 35 weeks gestation had 10 times the risk of those born at 40 weeks; and those born at 36 weeks had five times the risk of those born at 40 weeks gestation. Shapiro-Mendoza et al. (2008) further demonstrated that the proportion of babies with newborn morbidities increased with a greater number of maternal morbidities; 17.9% of late preterm infants had no reported maternal morbidities, 28.7% had at least one maternal morbidity reported, and 36.6% had two or more maternal morbidities reported. In comparison, full-term infants had 2.5%, 4.6%, and 7.6% for each number of maternal morbidities, respectively.

A study published in the *Journal of Perinatology* (Underwood, Danielson, & Gilbert, 2007) examined the cost and rates of rehospitalization of preterm infants (less than 36 weeks gestation) born in California from January 1992 through December 2000. Results showed that 13% of all babies born at 34 and 35 weeks gestation were readmitted to hospital within the first year of life, with 34-week-gestation babies incurring a cost of $64.3 million and 35-week-gestation babies incurring a cost of $92.9 million just in California.

LATE PRETERM BIRTH COMPLICATIONS

The short- and long-term complications of late preterm births have been well documented (Bérard, Le Tiec, & De Vera, 2012; Consortium on Safe Labor, 2010; Davis et al., 2011; Darnall, Ariagno, & Kinney, 2006; De Luca, Boulvain, Irion, Berner, & Pfister, 2009; Hunt, 2006; Lubow, How, Habli, Maxwell, & Sibai, 2009; Ma et al., 2009; Mally, Hendricks-Muñoz, & Bailey, 2012; McIntire & Leveno, 2008; Medoff Cooper et al., 2012; Raju et al., 2006; Shapiro-Mendoza et al., 2008; Wang, Dorer, Fleming, & Catlin, 2004). Short-term complications include feeding difficulties, jaundice, hypoglycemia, temperature instability, apnea, respiratory distress, hypotonia, increased risk of infection, and dehydration. Long-term complications include those associated with cognitive problems, school performance, behavior and psychiatric problems, increased risk for sudden infant death syndrome (SIDS) and, later on, reproductive problems (Cheong & Doyle, 2012; Huddy, Johnson, & Hope, 2001; Kirkegaard, Obel, Hedegaard, & Henriksen, 2006; Kramer et al., 2000; Lindström, Winbladh, Haglund, & Hjern, 2007; Moster, Lie, & Markestad, 2008; Morse, Zheng, Tang, & Roth, 2009; Saigal & Doyle, 2008; Swamy, Ostbye, &

Skjaerven, 2008). Hospital readmissions in the first few weeks after discharge are predominantly due to acute respiratory disease, hyperbilirubinemia, suspected sepsis, feeding difficulties, dehydration, and failure to thrive (Escobar et al., 2005; Gartner, 2001; Maisels & Kring, 1998; Raju et al., 2006; Underwood, Danielsen, & Gilbert, 2007).

EFFECTIVE BREASTFEEDING TO PREVENT COMPLICATIONS

Although long-term sequelae are multifaceted and lack a clear path of avoidance, short-term complications and hospital readmissions definitely can be decreased or eliminated by effective breastfeeding. Avoiding the common breastfeeding mistakes of not feeding often enough, assuming adequate transfer of breast milk when the infant appears satiated, improper positioning, delay of breastfeeding assistance to the late preterm infant, and delay or omission of maternal nipple stimulation and breast milk removal is imperative to effective breastfeeding in the late preterm population.

SUMMARY

Late preterm infants are babies born between 34 0/7 and 36 6/7 weeks gestation. Previously considered small full-term babies and treated as such, these babies have difficulties adapting to extra-uterine life. They have immature physiological functioning and are therefore at high risk for morbidities and mortality. Although in recent decades late preterm births have increased worldwide, medical professionals have come to realize that deliveries between 34 and 37 weeks gestation pose many risks to the baby, both immediately after birth and in the long term. Effective breastfeeding is the key to combating many complications, but successful breastfeeding is difficult to fully achieve with late preterm infants without proper education and early interventions.

TWO

Risk Factors for Late Preterm Births

COMMON CAUSES OF LATE PRETERM BIRTH

The reasons we are seeing a large increase in late preterm births are multifaceted. In the past, obstetricians may have been delivering these babies earlier than necessary because there was the assumption they would fare the same as full-term infants once the 36-week gestation mark was reached. As we have come to realize, this is not the case. Obstetricians are now more likely to wait for a longer gestation before elective deliveries are performed.

Maternal medical factors can lead to either spontaneous delivery of a late preterm infant or the need for medically indicated deliveries. These maternal morbidities can include preeclampsia, placental abruption, oligohydramnios, Rh disease, diabetes, chronic hypertension, asthma, cardiac disease, renal disease, and autoimmune disorders. Other maternal factors that have been cited as increasing the risk of delivering an infant prematurely include infertility treatments, increasing maternal age, multiple gestations, obesity, smoking, previous delivery of a premature infant, and maternal comorbid conditions (Blencowe, 2012; Cedergren, 2004; Cheong & Doyle, 2012; England, Benjamin, & Abenhaim, 2012; Loftin et al., 2010; Sibai, 2006; World Health Organization, 2012).

Fetal complications such as intrauterine growth retardation, congenital malformations, nonreassuring fetal test results, and premature rupture of membranes all contribute to premature deliveries (Loftin et al., 2010).

MATERNAL MEDICAL CONDITIONS THAT CAN RESULT IN LATE PRETERM DELIVERIES AND CREATE BREASTFEEDING CHALLENGES

Preeclampsia

Preeclampsia, also known as toxemia of pregnancy, is an abnormal condition of pregnancy that develops after 20 weeks gestation. It is characterized by the onset of acute hypertension and proteinuria, with or without pathologic edema. The global incidence of preeclampsia is estimated to be around 5% to 14% of all pregnancies.

Preeclampsia can be classified as mild or severe. With mild preeclampsia, physicians often opt to continue to monitor the mother until 37 weeks gestation, then deliver the infant to prevent further complications to both mother and baby. Prophylactic magnesium sulfate is usually given once the mother develops severe preeclampsia, because severe preeclampsia can lead to liver failure, renal failure, disseminated intravascular coagulation (DIC), and central nervous system abnormalities in the mother (Lim & Steinberg, 2011), as well as ischemic encephalopathy, growth retardation, and various sequelae of premature births in the infants. HELLP syndrome, which gets its name from its characteristic symptoms of *h*emolysis, *e*levated *l*iver enzyme level, and *l*ow *p*latelet count, may also be a result of severe preeclampsia. If associated seizures develop, the condition has progressed to eclampsia.

Magnesium sulfate given to the mother can have negative effects on the newborn, including respiratory depression, hypotonia, lethargy, and poor suck reflex (Verklan & Walden, 2010). Severe preeclampsia, eclampsia, and HELLP syndrome can all result in the delivery of late preterm infants. Magnesium administration can have compounding negative effects on the neurologically immature late preterm infant, who is already at a breastfeeding disadvantage.

Placental Abruption

Placental abruption is the separation of the placenta from the wall of the uterus before the baby is delivered. Direct causes, although rare, can be from injury to the abdomen or sudden loss of uterine volume, such as seen after a first twin is delivered. Known risk factors include blood clotting disorders, cigarette smoking, cocaine use, excess alcohol consumption, history of previous placental abruption, diabetes, high blood pressure, increased uterine distention, older mother, large number of past deliveries, premature rupture of membranes, and uterine fibroids (Animated Dissection of Anatomy for Medicine Medical Encyclopedia, 2013). Placental abruption occurs in about 1 out of 150 deliveries. The mother can exhibit signs of shock, and the fetus may exhibit an abnormal heart rate. If the mother and fetus stabilize without a large loss of blood, emergency delivery of the fetus is postponed. A large placental abruption can result in the delivery of a late preterm baby who may be hypovolemic and listless.

Oligohydramnios

Oligohydramnios is a condition of decreased amniotic fluid volume. The earlier it occurs in pregnancy, the poorer the prognosis for the fetus. Before 22 weeks it can result in major congenital malformations and pulmonary hypoplasia. In the second trimester it can result in pulmonary hypoplasia, fetal compression syndrome, and amniotic banding. In late preterm gestation, the fetus may present with intrauterine growth retardation (IUGR). Oligohydramnios is often associated with abnormal fetal heart rate, meconium-stained fluid, and increased incidence of cesarean delivery (Baxter, Sehdev, & Breckenridge, 2012). When meconium is present in the amniotic fluid at birth, the baby is often subjected to increased oral suctioning, and the suctioning itself plus the irritation from the meconium can result in the infant being unwilling to swallow, leading to feeding aversion. The medications used during the cesarean section can cause sleepiness in the baby, and the extra fluid the mother receives during the surgery can result in nipple or areolar edema, making latching during breastfeeding difficult.

Rh Disease

Merriam-Webster's Medical Desk Dictionary (2013) defines Rh disease, also known as erythroblastosis fetalis, as a hemolytic disease of the fetus and newborn, characterized by an increase in circulating erythroblasts and jaundice. It occurs when an Rh-negative mother produces antibodies to an antigen in the blood of an Rh-positive fetus, which cross the placenta and destroy fetal red blood cells. This resulting jaundice can require phototherapy, supplementation, or intravenous fluid therapy, all with negative effects on breastfeeding.

Diabetes

Poorly regulated maternal diabetes, exposing the fetus to prolonged elevated glucose levels, can result in chronic fetal hyperinsulinemia. This hyperinsulinemia triggers increased oxygen consumption and metabolism, leading to chronic intrauterine tissue hypoxia. The hypoxia can cause alterations in myelination and cortical connectivity in the fetus's brain, which can profoundly affect the neurodevelopment of the infant (Capra, Tezza, Mazzei, & Boner, 2013). The late preterm infant is already at a neurological disadvantage, having an immature brain that can lead to poor breastfeeding outcomes, and this resultant hypoxia further decreases the chances of breastfeeding success.

In a study of 893 late preterm infants, maternal gestational diabetes was found to be commonly associated with hypoglycemia (Hellmeyer et al., 2012); other studies have indicated that maternal gestational diabetes exposes neonates born after 34 weeks to an increased risk of severe neonatal respiratory failure (Gouyon et al., 2010; Vignoles et al., 2011).

Chronic Hypertension

Chronic, untreated hypertension during pregnancy carries an increased risk for having a low-birth-weight infant, preterm birth, and an infant that is small for gestational age. Left untreated, hypertension also poses a greater maternal risk of developing preeclampsia, placental abruption, and gestational diabetes (James & Nelson-Piercy, 2004). In a study to determine the effects of several antihypertensive drugs, Su et al. (2013) demonstrated that, compared to treatment with other types of antihypertensive drugs, women who received vasodilators for their chronic hypertension exhibited the highest risk of having low-birth-weight infants, preterm births, and infants who are small for gestational age.

Other treatments of hypertension include alpha-agonists, beta-blockers, calcium channel blockers, and diuretics. Su et al. (2013) point out several conflicting studies aimed at addressing the use of antihypertensives in pregnant women.

Asthma

According to Capra et al. (2013), nearly 10% of pregnant women are affected by asthma. Exacerbations of asthma during pregnancy are associated with low birth weight, and inadequate control of symptoms can lead to an 11% incidence of preterm delivery, compared with a 6% incidence with well-controlled cases. This incidence of preterm deliveries increases to 16% if hospitalization is required for control of symptoms.

Cardiac Disease

In a retrospective study by Ouyang, Khairy, Fernandes, Landzberg, and Economy (2010), 112 pregnancies of women with congenital heart disease were examined in terms of adverse obstetrical events. The most common adverse event was preterm delivery, followed by postpartum hemorrhage. Siu et al. (2001) examined data from a study of 562 women with cardiac disease and found preterm births to be the leading adverse event as well.

Renal Disease

Renal disease, which can present with anything from proteinuria to the need for dialysis, can result in increased numbers of late preterm births. Shahir, Briggs, Katsoulis, and Levidiotis (2013), who reviewed data from 49 pregnancies of women with renal disease that required dialysis, noted a preeclampsia rate of 19.4% (as noted above, preeclampsia increases the risk of late preterm delivery), 53.4% preterm births, 65% low birth weight, and 35% very low birth weight. The low birth weight correlated with prematurity. Xie, Zhang, Wang, Wang, and Zhang (2012) analyzed data from 48 patients and found 15 of the 48 (31%) had preterm deliveries and 11 of the 48 babies (23%) were small for gestational age.

Autoimmune Disorders

An array of autoimmune diseases, if uncontrolled, are associated with an increased incidence of preterm births and infants with low birth weight. Johnson, Petri, Witter, and Repke (1995) reported that the rate of premature rupture of membranes was higher in women with systemic lupus erythematosus (SLE) than in the control group without SLE, and the premature rupture of membranes leads to an increase in preterm births. In a review by Adams Waldorf and Nelson (2008), the authors stated that untreated thyroid disease could lead to low-birth-weight infants and preterm deliveries.

Infertility Treatment

The use of fertility treatments is associated with the trend to delay childbearing. In 2002, more than 50% of women seeking infertility treatment in the United States were 35 years of age or older (Institute of Medicine, 2007), which is usually considered to be advanced maternal age in the United States. In a summary of assisted reproductive technology (ART) use during 2009, Sunderam et al. (2012) found that a total of 146,244 ART procedures were reported to the Centers for Disease Control and Prevention (CDC), as mandated by law. As a result of these procedures, 60,190 infants were delivered. Of these infants, 47% were multiple births, compared with 3% of infants among the general population; 32% were low birth weight, compared with 8% in the general population; and 33.4% were born between 32 and 37 weeks gestation, compared with 12.2% of the general population.

Advanced Maternal Age

Carolan, Davey, Biro, and Kealy (2013) examined data collected from pregnant women of very advanced maternal age (45 years or older) and compared those 217 women with 48,909 pregnant women ages 30 to 34 years to determine the maternal and perinatal outcomes of these pregnancies. The older women had an increased risk of gestational diabetes and antepartum hemorrhage, as well as preterm birth between 32 and 36 weeks, having a low-birth-weight infant, and having a baby who is small for gestational age. Kenny et al. (2013) performed a population-based cohort study consisting of 215,344 births and found that women who were 40 years or older at delivery were at increased risk of stillborn births, preterm births, macrosomia, and caesarean delivery.

Twins or Higher-Level Multiples

Preterm delivery is the most serious complication of pregnancies with multiples. Kurdi, Mesleh, Al-Hakeem, Khashoggi, and Khalifa (2004) demonstrated that premature labor in multiple-gestation pregnancies was seven times higher than in singleton pregnancies, and 49% of multiples were delivered by cesarean, compared to 14% of singletons.

Obesity

The World Health Organization (2013) classifies body weight based on body mass index (BMI), as follows:

- Underweight: BMI 18.50 or less
- Normal weight: BMI 18.50 to 24.99
- Overweight: BMI 25.00 to 29.99

- Obese class I: BMI 30.00 to 34.99
- Obese class II: BMI 35.00 to 39.99
- Obese class III: BMI 40 or greater

A retrospective study by Scott-Pillai, Spence, Cardwell, Hunter, and Holmes (2013) assessed the prevalence of overweight and obesity and the impact of BMI on maternal and neonatal outcomes by studying data from 30,298 singleton pregnancies over an 8-year period. Compared to women of normal weight, women who were overweight or obese had a significantly increased risk for hypertensive disorders, gestational diabetes, induction of labor, caesarean delivery, and postpartum hemorrhage. Women in obese classes II and III were at even greater risk for these same problems. Women in obese class III were at increased risk of preterm delivery and stillbirth and of having infants who required admission to the neonatal intensive care unit (NICU).

Using retrospective analysis of data from 287,213 singleton deliveries, another group of researchers (Sebire et al., 2001) found the same results in overweight and obese class I women and also found an increased risk for preeclampsia among this group. However, in overweight and obese women, they found a decreased risk for delivery before 32 weeks and, unfortunately, decreased breastfeeding outcomes at discharge.

Smoking

Smoking during pregnancy has been associated with reductions in birth weight of up to 642 grams (Wang et al., 2002) and decreased in-utero brain growth (Herrmann, King, & Weitzman, 2008). A prospective cohort study of 2,504 women was used to compare pregnancy outcomes among women who stopped smoking in early pregnancy (before 15 weeks gestation) and those who either did not smoke in pregnancy or continued to smoke (McCowan et al., 2009). There were no differences in rates of spontaneous preterm births or small-for-gestational-age infants between nonsmokers and stopped smokers, but current smokers had a 10% higher risk for spontaneous preterm birth and 17% higher risk for small-for-gestational-age infants than stopped smokers. Further review of data by Herrmann et al. (2008) revealed that smoking and secondhand smoke can cause markedly increased rates of neurological impairment to an exposed fetus and newborn, including increased rates of behavior problems such as irritability, oppositional defiant behavior, conduct disorders, and attention-deficit/hyperactivity disorder (ADHD).

Previous Delivery of a Premature Infant

Using a historical cohort study, Simonsen et al. (2013) were able to determine that a history of preterm birth increased the risk for a recurrent preterm birth by 21% of second births; if the first or second birth was premature, the risk of a third birth being premature was 22%. Risk factors for recurrence of preterm births included short intervals between pregnancies, underweight prepregnant BMI, preexisting maternal medical conditions, previous preterm birth at 28 to 32 weeks gestation, presence of fetal anomalies, and young maternal age.

OTHER RISK FACTORS FOR LATE PRETERM BIRTHS

Dekker et al. (2012) identified independent risk factors for preterm births (< 37 weeks). Studying 3,234 healthy nulliparous women with singleton pregnancies, the researchers divided the results into spontaneous preterm births with intact membranes and spontaneous preterm births after premature rupture of membranes (PROM). They concluded that spontaneous preterm births with intact membranes were associated with shorter cervical length, abnormal uterine Doppler flow, maternal prepregnancy use of marijuana, lack of overall feeling of well-being, being of Caucasian ethnicity, having a mother with diabetes and/or a history of preeclampsia, and having a family history of low-birth-weight babies. Independent risk factors for spontaneous preterm birth after PROM included short cervical length, short stature, mother not being firstborn in the family, longer time to conceive, not waking up at night during pregnancy, hormonal fertility treatment (excluding clomiphene), mild hypertension, family history of recurring gestational diabetes, and low BMI (< 20). Interestingly, having a BMI less than 20 nearly doubled the risk for spontaneous preterm birth.

SUMMARY

Although many factors contribute to the birth of late preterm infants, taking precautions to eliminate unnecessary deliveries of infants before term is paramount. Technological advances, increased maternal age, and subsequent increased maternal morbidities are taking their toll on the rates of late preterm deliveries. Although many risk factors cannot be eliminated, reducing the ones that can will help to slow the rise in the late preterm population.

THREE

Immature Neurological Development and Hypotonia

There is strong evidence that supports a relationship between gestational age at birth and degree of brain maturation. Lack of brain control predisposes the late preterm infant to altered sleep states, hypotonia, and decreased response to rooting reflexes, among other things, all of which can lead to poor breastfeeding.

RESEARCH INTO THE BRAIN OF THE LATE PRETERM INFANT

Although once considered to be just small full-term babies, and because of the lack of treatment and monitoring given to them based on this assumption, late preterm infants have now proven themselves as a separate class of infants as a result of their increased risk for serious complications. The laid-back approach to their care has had serious long-term consequences, which the medical profession has now come to realize.

In terms of brain growth, it's not merely the size of the brain that is different; the functionality of the brain differs in earlier gestation. As the fetus progresses to term, brain size increases, maturation of many processes occurs, and the brain becomes adequately functional for a term infant to thrive and breastfeed successfully.

BRAIN MATURATION PROCESS

Davis et al. (2011) conducted a study to determine if children's brain development benefits from longer gestations. Magnetic resonance imaging (MRI) scans were performed on 100 children between the ages of 6 and 10; 67 of the children were born at term and 33 of them were born between 28 and 39 weeks, all of whom were healthy at delivery, did not require mechanical ventilation, and were free from any brain injury. The MRI scans indicated that there were regionally specific incremental increases in gray matter as gestation progressed toward term. An increase in gray matter volume increases the effectiveness of all spinal reflexes. The researchers were able to conclude that among healthy, low-risk populations, shortened gestation has persisting influences on neurological development.

Disruptions to brain development associated with shorter gestation, as with late preterm births, increase the risk for the development of behavioral and psychological dysfunction throughout the life span. Although late preterm babies are at an advantage over less mature babies, they do have a slight disadvantage when compared with their full-term counterparts (Schothorst, Swaab-Barneveld, & van Engeland, 2007). Lack of brain maturation also leaves them susceptible to difficulties adapting to the stressors of extra-uterine life.

Scher, Johnson, Ludington, and Loparo (2011) describe this brain immaturity as "brain dysmaturity" in late preterm infants. Their research used electroencephalographic (EEG) studies to determine if there were differences in sleep between late preterm infants and term infants. They identified eight late preterm infants who were clinically asymptomatic throughout the study period and not treated for severe respiratory distress syndrome, sepsis, encephalopathy, or seizures and compared them with eight similar full-term infants. Late preterm infants showed fewer arousals and more immature or shorter sleep cycles. Scher et al. (2011) demonstrated six of seven measures that differentiated late preterm infants from full-term infants in terms of neuronal networks. They concluded that maturation of integrated autonomic brainstem function is delayed in late preterm infants compared to term infants and that environmental stress alters sleep expression. These results could have a huge impact on breastfeeding late preterm infants.

Darnall, Ariangno, and Kinney (2006) also demonstrated that there are dramatic and nonlinear developmental changes in the brainstem as the infant approaches term gestation and that lack of maturation in the late preterm infant corresponds to altered sleep patterns. Studying 78 premature and term newborns with postconceptual ages of 29 to 41 weeks, Hüppi et al. (1998) demonstrated a linear increase in total brain tissue volume of 22 mL per week. More astonishing was their determination that absolute volume of myelinated white matter increased fivefold from 35 to 41 weeks and that one third of brain growth occurs between 35 and 41 weeks gestation.

Perhaps Volpe (2009) gives us the best overall picture of the differences in brain development between term babies and babies born late preterm. Multiple developmental events involving brain maturation take place between 24 and 40 weeks gestation, which leaves any preterm baby predisposed to increased risk of brain injury. In the absence of injury, the cerebral cortex is involved in dendritic development and extensive refinement of synapsed afferent axonal terminals. A fourfold increase in cerebral cortical volume from 28 to 40 weeks gestation has been documented. This expansion of the cerebral cortex corresponds to an increased cortical surface area and rapid gyral development. In addition, the cerebellum increases in volume three times from 28 weeks to 40 weeks, and with its increase comes an increase in cortical surface area as well as neuronal proliferation and migration.

Zanin et al. (2011) used magnetic resonance diffusion tensor imaging tractography to distinguish between the main stages of white matter maturation in normal fetuses. White matter, involved in the myelination of the spinal cord, is composed of myelinated axons. Myelin insulates the neural circuitry; prevents the leakage of current; and enables rapid, efficient transmission of nerve impulses (Verklan & Walden, 2010). Zanin et al. (2011) demonstrated that myelination occurs from weeks 35 through 39 and that a mature, visually evoked response does not occur until 39 weeks gestation, proving the limitations of the late preterm infant's brain. Larsen and Stensaas (2003) discuss the corticospinal tract just starting to myelinate at 36 weeks. These studies prove that late preterm babies will likely have difficulty reacting to their extra-uterine environment, with negative effects on the success of breastfeeding.

Finally, Marsh, Gerber, and Peterson (2008) used histological and postmortem findings to study brain development in relation to understanding childhood neuropsychiatric disorders. Their research concludes that synaptogenesis peaks after 34 weeks gestation at a rate of 40,000 new synapses per second, and continues in postnatal life. That number of new synapses is astounding. It is no wonder a late preterm infant's brain functioning is so much more immature than a term infant's brain function.

POOR ADAPTATION TO EXTRA-UTERINE LIFE

From these studies, we can determine that late preterm infants most likely will display less mature spinal reflexes; have decreased synapse transmission and, therefore, decreased purposeful movements; have different sleep cycles, which are apparent by less awake time; are more susceptible to difficulties adapting to stimuli; and are more prone to brain injury and neurological disturbances. Hypoglycemia, hypothermia, infection, and hyperbilirubinemia can all alter the intended path of neurological development in late preterm infants because the myelin coating that protects the nervous system is undeveloped.

It is well documented that late preterm infants have difficulty adapting to extra-uterine life (Cheng, Kaimal, Bruckner, Halloron, & Caughey, 2011; Dong & Yu, 2011; Engle, Tomashek, & Wallman, 2007; Hubbard, Stellwagen, & Wolf, 2007; Loftin et al., 2010; Radtke, 2011; Raju, Higgins, Stark, & Leveno, 2006; Wang, Dorer, Fleming, & Catlin, 2004). These babies often exhibit hypotonia, are very sleepy, and are poor feeders, all of which contribute to poor breastfeeding outcomes. The development of coordinated feeding follows a chronological and predictable pattern in late preterm infants (Hunt, 2006), suggesting that neurodevelopmental maturation, and not learned behavior or experience, dictates the progression of successful breastfeeding.

HOW THE IMMATURE BRAIN AFFECTS BREASTFEEDING

The most frustrating aspect of immature brain maturation in late preterm infants is likely the lack of time the baby is awake or remains awake for feedings. Because late preterm infants have longer periods of sleep and shorter periods of wakeful time than their full-term counterparts, mothers must be able to identify very early feeding cues and act upon those cues immediately. Even a delay of a few minutes can cause the baby to fall back to sleep without breastfeeding. Waiting for the late preterm baby to become fully awake is counterproductive because these babies don't often exhibit full wakefulness, except after the initial birth, until closer to term. Thinking that the baby will soon be hungry and wake up to feed has proven to have harmful consequences.

Constant skin-to-skin contact helps the baby to smell the breast and be more likely to wake and breastfeed while also encouraging more vigilance from the mother to watch for early hunger cues. While the baby is breastfeeding, a conscientious attempt to keep the baby awake and feeding well must be made. Breast compressions allow colostrum or breast milk to be pushed to the tip of the nipple, providing a continual taste to the baby and encouraging continued suckling without excess expenditure of energy. Babies tend to pause between suckling bursts, and if the pause is prolonged more than a couple of seconds, the late preterm infant has the potential to fall asleep or forget what he or she was doing, so again vigilance on the part of the mother to keep the baby suckling is essential. Even when babies appear to be asleep, they often will suckle if given the opportunity. Don't assume that because the eyes are closed the mouth won't work.

HOW HYPOTONIA AFFECTS BREASTFEEDING SUCCESS

Because of hypotonia, it is often difficult to position late preterm infants in a fully supported fashion. Dangling arms or legs interrupt the reflex pathways, and late preterm infants are less likely to have enough synapses firing well enough to focus their energy on breastfeeding. Hypotonia makes late preterm infants much more prone to flexion of their head and neck, causing difficulties with breathing, sucking, and swallowing, and predisposing them to increased energy consumption, early fatigue, regurgitation, and respiratory distress. Ensuring proper positioning with complete support of the whole baby helps to overcome these challenges. Hypotonia also plays a part in weak suckling and poor latch.

DECREASED REFLEXES INTERFERE WITH BREASTFEEDING

Lack of brain maturation corresponds to decreased reflexes, including rooting reflexes, which are most prominent at 40 weeks gestation. Therefore, late preterm infants may not respond to attempts to entice them to latch like full-term infants will. This typically results in the baby failing to open his or her mouth appropriately when normal rooting stimuli are used, such as touching the baby's chin to the mother's breast or rubbing the mother's nipple gently from the baby's nose to his or her chin. Placing your fingers on the baby's cheeks during latching or feeding can further inhibit breastfeeding by causing disruption in the normal rooting reflexes, because the baby then has to identify the difference between the true nipple in his or her mouth and the perceived nipple touching the cheek. When this happens, late preterm infants will often stop suckling altogether and may fall back asleep. Therefore, other methods of stimulating the baby to suck besides tapping the cheek should be utilized in the late preterm population.

DECREASED PURPOSEFUL MOVEMENTS

The lack of complete myelination decreases synaptic firings in the brain, making it difficult for the late preterm infant to do anything with purpose. Therefore, even if the baby latches, the mother's soft, pliable nipple may not be enough of a stimulus to initiate or maintain suckling as a result of the lack of efficient transmission of nerve impulses. In this case, a nipple shield is warranted and encouraged because it fills the mouth, providing more contact between the nipple and the tongue and mouth, increasing the chances of complete transmission of impulses by increasing synaptic firing.

EXCESS STRESS FROM EXTERNAL STIMULATION

Decreased amounts of gray and white matter and decreased surface area of the brain, as evidenced by insufficient gyri and sulci, affect the late preterm infant's ability to respond appropriately to normal extrauterine stressors. Motion, noise, touch, and light may all cause the baby to withdraw or shut down, as a mechanism to preserve necessary brain functioning. Each baby will have a unique threshold for how much of these stressors he or she can withstand, and at certain times an infant might be able to withstand more than at other times. Breastfeeding involves motion to properly position the infant and touch for latching and suckling, as well as skin-to-skin contact. Often this is all the late preterm infant can endure, so care must be taken not to overstimulate the baby with added motion such as rocking chairs, extra touch such as stroking, or noise and excess light during breastfeeding. Although mothers are often tempted to talk to their babies while breastfeeding, late preterm infants may not be able to effectively breastfeed while being bombarded with all these stimuli.

SUMMARY

Understanding the brain's development is the key to understanding the challenges late preterm infants face with breastfeeding. As evidenced by research, brain maturation occurs in stages and late preterm infants have much less brain volume and much less efficient functioning than their full-term counterparts. This lack of maturation increases the risk for brain injury as well as developmental and psychological dysfunction. Lack of brain maturity can result in hypotonia, sleepiness, lack of appropriate reflexes, and the inability to properly respond to stimuli, all of which result in poor breastfeeding outcomes. By understanding the progression of brain maturation, health care professionals will be better equipped to help these late preterm infants with successful breastfeeding. Teaching parents about the brain maturation process will better enable them to understand the progression of breastfeeding success and will likely curb their feelings of inadequacy in feeding the late preterm infant.

FOUR

Temperature Instability, Hypoglycemia, and Increased Metabolism

Temperature instability, hypoglycemia, and increased metabolism are all common conditions experienced by the late preterm infant. Each condition on its own creates issues with homeostasis and adaptation to extra-uterine life, but when combined, as is often the case with late preterm infants, their consequences can be exponential. The need for early, effective, and frequent breastfeeding is paramount to prevent complications related to all three of these medical challenges.

THE IMPORTANCE OF THERMOREGULATION IN THE LATE PRETERM INFANT

Temperature stability, or thermoregulation, is especially important to maintain in late preterm infants because hypothermia can lead to increased oxygenation requirements, hypoglycemia, and jaundice; all of which have a significant impact on breastfeeding success. Hyperthermia, on the other hand, is often caused by completely unavoidable factors such as overheating from a radiant warmer, overdressing, or leaving a baby dressed and wrapped in a blanket during breastfeeding. Hyperthermia can undermine breastfeeding success by causing irritability, lethargy, cardiac arrhythmias, and dehydration. Both hyperthermia and hypothermia can be symptoms of sepsis in an infant, so maintaining temperature homeostasis is important in ruling out sepsis and preventing unnecessary procedures, pain to the infant, separation of mother and baby, and increased medical costs.

THERMOREGULATION OF THE ADULT

When an adult is cold, an autonomic response to the cold stress is exhibited by shivering. The shivering helps increase core temperature. Likewise, increased metabolic activity, such as exercise, helps to increase core temperature. Sweating helps to cool us down when core temperatures become higher than normal. Neither of these autonomic responses to heat or cold is present in the newborn, so regulation of temperature becomes much more difficult and complex for them.

BROWN FAT: ITS ROLE IN THERMOREGULATION

Fetuses begin producing a specialized tissue called brown fat at 26 to 28 weeks gestation, and stores continue to increase throughout pregnancy and until 3 to 5 weeks postnatally (Verklan & Walden, 2010). Brown fat is highly vascularized, which gives the fat its characteristic brown color and serves to conduct heat into the baby's circulation. It is typically located at the nape of the neck, interscapular region, axillae, groin, and around the kidneys and adrenals. When a baby's skin becomes cold, afferent nerves send messages to the heat regulation center in the hypothalamus, triggering efferent nerves supplying the brown fat to stimulate release of noradrenalin (Mishra & Pati, 2004). This release of noradrenalin results in oxidation of triglycerides to glycerol and fatty acids, and the fatty acids are consumed locally, resulting in the generation of heat. The brown fat becomes heated, and the heat is distributed through the bloodstream to various body parts of the newborn, warming the baby.

SUBCUTANEOUS FAT

Subcutaneous fat, also known as white fat, accounts for 16% of body fat in neonates and plays a role in insulation (Verklan & Walden, 2010). Term newborn infants have approximately three times the surface-area-to-weight ratio as adults, and preterm infants have approximately five times the surface-area-to-weight ratio. Heat transfer from the neonate's organs to the skin surface is increased because of the decreased amounts of subcutaneous fat and increased surface-area-to-weight ratio. This transfer of heat results in increased heat loss to the environment, and the large surface-area-to-weight ratio results in increased transepidermal water loss as a result of evaporation.

DISADVANTAGES CAUSING HYPOTHERMIA IN THE LATE PRETERM INFANT

Late preterm infants have less time in utero to attain fat stores and therefore are born with less brown fat and less subcutaneous fat, resulting in decreased ability to maintain temperature homeostasis. There simply is not enough brown fat to warm the body. Late preterm infants have a larger surface-area-to-weight ratio, leading to greater transfer of heat to the environment and greater evaporative heat loss. Although term infants are better able to decrease heat loss from exposed body surfaces by assuming a flexed position, a late preterm infant usually is more hypotonic and assumes a more extended position, resulting in increased surface subject to heat loss. Late preterm infants are also at a disadvantage compared to full-term infants because of poor breastfeeding, resulting in the inability to consume enough calories to provide nutrients for thermogenesis.

HOW HYPOTHERMIA LEADS TO HYPOGLYCEMIA, INCREASED OXYGEN CONSUMPTION, AND JAUNDICE

The process of triglyceride oxidation to convert brown fat to heat requires increased oxygen and glucose consumption. This increased oxygen consumption can put further strain on an already compromised infant at risk for respiratory distress, such as the late preterm infant. Increased oxygen consumption can lead to increased lactic acid production, resulting in metabolic acidosis, which can lead to pulmonary vasoconstriction and decreased blood flow to vital organs (Verklan & Walden, 2010).

Maintenance of normal temperature helps infants regulate energy consumption. Anaerobic heat production increases glucose consumption, possibly leading to hypoglycemia, which is already a common complication exhibited by late preterm infants. Hypoglycemia can then, in turn, cause hypothermia because there is not enough glucose to use for heat energy.

Hypothermia can also lead to increased jaundice, as metabolism of brown fat releases fatty acids that compete with bilirubin for albumin-binding sites (Verklan & Walden, 2010).

RESEARCH CONFIRMING THE LATE PRETERM INFANT'S RISK FOR HYPOTHERMIA

Hellmeyer et al. (2012) evaluated neonatal outcomes of 893 late preterm infants and found that gestational diabetes of the mother leads to a reduced risk of hypothermia compared to late preterm infants whose mothers did not have diabetes.

Tsai et al. (2012) compared 6,507 term infants with 914 late preterm infants and found the risk for temperature instability for late preterm infants was much higher than in term infants (0.4% vs. 0.05%).

Wang, Dorer, Fleming, and Catlin (2004) analyzed data from 90 late preterm infants and 95 full-term infants and found late preterm infants to be much more likely to exhibit temperature instability than full-term infants (10% vs. 0%).

WHAT IS HYPOGLYCEMIA?

The definition of hypoglycemia, besides that of low blood glucose concentration, remains somewhat elusive, because physicians hesitate to assign an absolute number for acceptable blood glucose concentrations in newborns. The American Academy of Pediatrics (2011) provides a clinical report with practical guidelines for screening and management of hypoglycemia, which states that current evidence does not support a specific concentration of glucose considered to be either normal or abnormal. Clinically significant neonatal hypoglycemia reflects an imbalance between glucose intake, glucose production, and glucose use by the body (Verklan & Walden, 2010) and is influenced by factors such as postconceptual age, adequacy of gluconeogenic (glucose-producing) pathways, general health status, and presence or absence of symptoms. Medical management of hypoglycemia should be based on a combination of all these factors.

INFANTS AT RISK FOR HYPOGLYCEMIA

According to the American Academy of Pediatrics (2011), neonatal hypoglycemia occurs most commonly in infants who are small for their gestational age, infants born to mothers who have diabetes, and late preterm infants. Further risk factors for hypoglycemia (Verklan & Walden, 2010) that increase the rate of metabolism and decrease energy stores include:

- Asphyxia
- Increased work of breathing
- Cold stress
- Sepsis

EVIDENCE OF INCREASED RISK OF HYPOGLYCEMIA AMONG LATE PRETERM INFANTS

Several researchers have found a correlation between late preterm infants and the increased risk of hypoglycemia. A descriptive analysis of data (Medoff Cooper et al., 2012) from 14 hospitals across the United States and Canada indicated that more than half of the 802 late preterm infants experienced hypoglycemia.

Wang et al. (2004), in their data collection from 90 late preterm infants and 95 term infants, found, among other things, that late preterm infants were much more likely to exhibit hypoglycemia than were full-term infants (15.6% vs. 5.3%).

Engle, Tomashek, and Wallman (2007) describe hypoglycemia as something that can affect fasting newborn infants of any gestational age in response to the abrupt loss of maternal glucose supply after birth. They further state that the incidence of hypoglycemia is inversely proportional to gestational age; that is, the lower the gestational age, the more likely hypoglycemia is to occur.

Hellmeyer et al. (2012) evaluated outcomes of 893 late preterm infants and found that gestational diabetes of the mother was more commonly associated with infant hypoglycemia, and that those infants born by cesarean section were at a higher risk of hypoglycemia than those who were born vaginally.

SYMPTOMS OF HYPOGLYCEMIA

Symptoms of hypoglycemia can mimic a wide range of clinical conditions common in sick neonates (American Academy of Pediatrics, 2011; Verklan & Walden, 2010) and can include:

- Tremors, jitteriness, irritability, exaggerated Moro reflex, seizures
- High-pitched or weak cry
- Cyanosis, apnea, tachypnea

- Hypotonia, lethargy
- Hypothermia, temperature instability
- Poor feeding
- Eye rolling

Some of these symptoms of hypoglycemia are commonly seen as a manifestation of late preterm infants' immature neurological, immunological, and respiratory systems, and it may be difficult to differentiate between normal late preterm behavior and hypoglycemia without performing glucose testing.

THE ROLE OF BROWN FAT IN THE METABOLIC PATHWAY

As discussed earlier with temperature instability, late preterm infants are often lacking the deposits of brown fat that term infants acquire in late gestation. These brown fat deposits, which make term babies appear chubby, are used in the initial days after birth to maintain temperature and to supply the infant with energy until breastfeeding becomes successful and the baby can obtain all of his or her nutrition from breast milk.

In a term infant, this brown fat is broken down into fatty acids and glycerol. Fatty acids are responsible for increasing blood flow to the body for warmth and temperature stability, and glycerol is used in the gluconeogenesis pathway to produce energy and maintain glucose homeostasis.

HEPATIC GLYCOGEN HELPS MAINTAIN GLUCOSE HOMEOSTASIS

Immediately after delivery and the cutting of the umbilical cord, the baby no longer receives glucose from his or her mother. At this point, hepatic glycogen stores are mobilized (glycogenolysis) to provide a continuing source of glucose to the brain. Up to 90% of hepatic glycogen stores are used up in the first 3 hours of life in a healthy term infant (Verklan & Walden, 2010).

HOW GLYCOGENOLYSIS AND GLUCONEOGENESIS AFFECT THE LATE PRETERM INFANT

Because of the decreased incubation time in utero, late preterm infants have much less brown fat and reduced hepatic glycogen stores. In addition, the immaturity of the liver decreases their ability to convert stored glycogen (Verklan & Walden, 2010).

Human organs, especially the brain, are primarily dependent on glucose as their major energy source. Infants have a much higher brain-to-body-weight ratio than adults, and in late preterm infants this is even more pronounced. Cerebral glucose utilization accounts for 90% of the newborn's total glucose consumption (Verkaln & Walden, 2010).

The infant brain initially metabolizes lactate, which is present in abundance to provide continued fuel to the brain even though glucose concentrations are low. Within the first 3 or 4 hours after birth, glucose has begun mobilizing from hepatic and brown fat stores in healthy full-term infants, but in late preterm infants who do not have the hepatic glycogen stores or the brown fat stores, this glucose is rapidly depleted. Without early, effective breastfeeding, hypoglycemia and its resultant morbidities can quickly ensue.

INCREASED ENERGY METABOLISM

With decreased glucose available for energy, the body uses alternate fuels such as ketone bodies, lactic acid, free fatty acids, and glycerol, if they are available, to ensure enough glucose for the brain. This increases metabolism, oxygen consumption, and insensible water loss.

HOW INCREASED METABOLISM AFFECTS THE LATE PRETERM INFANT

Increased metabolism burns extra calories, something that late preterm infants simply cannot afford. This leads to hypoglycemia as well as excess weight loss in the late preterm infant.

The increased oxygen consumption associated with increased metabolism further predisposes late preterm infants to respiratory distress, often resulting in tachypnea.

The insensible water loss attributed to increased metabolism predisposes the late preterm infant to dehydration.

SUMMARY

Temperature instability has several negative effects on a late preterm infant, increasing the risk for other morbidities and leading to unsuccessful breastfeeding. It is imperative that we maintain a neutral thermal environment for the late preterm infant, stressing the importance of this to parents, teaching about both hypothermia and hyperthermia. The most effective strategy to maintain the late preterm infant's temperature is by keeping constant skin-to-skin contact of mother and baby, as outlined in Chapter 13, "Decrease Stimuli and Energy Expenditure." A well-educated mother will attempt to maintain a neutral thermal environment for her baby, but if not educated about the effects of both cold stress and overheating, she will feel responsible and guilty for causing increased complications in her already compromised infant.

Although hypoglycemia in itself is not a disease, the symptoms of hypoglycemia are precursors to the deterioration of the infant's health. Hypoglycemia should *always* be anticipated in late preterm infants, and steps should be taken to avoid unnecessary increases in glucose demand. A neutral thermal environment should be maintained, and early, frequent, and effective breastfeeding should be initiated, using the strategies such as continuous skin-to-skin contact, decreasing stimuli and energy expenditure, proper positioning, and breast compressions, all of which are presented in the second part of this book.

Proper education for the parents about the importance of decreasing energy demands of the baby is essential for eliminating external causes of hypoglycemia. Appropriate methods to combat this complication should be immediately initiated at birth, and assistance to the parents to maintain glucose homeostasis should be provided throughout the hospital stay.

FIVE

Hyperbilirubinemia

WHAT IS BILIRUBIN?

Bilirubin is primarily the metabolic end product of the breakdown of hemoglobin in old red blood cells (Verklan & Walden, 2010). Jaundice is the yellow pigment that is visible in the skin and the whites of the eyes when levels of bilirubin rise. In adults, the bilirubin formed from old red blood cells does not usually cause jaundice because the liver metabolizes it and the gut rids the body of it. However, infants often become jaundiced from the breakdown of red blood cells in the first few days after birth for several reasons.

First, the liver enzyme that breaks down the bilirubin, uridine diphosphate glucuronyl transferase (UGT; Hubbard, Stellwagen, & Wolf, 2007), is relatively immature, with lower activity with decreasing gestational age.

Second, newborns have more red blood cells than do adults and newborn red blood cells don't live as long as adult red blood cells, so breakdown occurs more frequently (Newman, 2009).

Third, an infant's bilirubin level is dependent on a balance of bilirubin production and elimination. Infants with impaired hemolytic processes, G6PD deficiency, polycythemia, or bruising may have more red cell breakdown and increased bilirubin production (Hubbard et al., 2007). Newborns typically don't feed well in the first few days, so elimination of bilirubin from the gut is slow.

High levels of bilirubin (hyperbilirubinemia) can cause kernicterus, also known as acute bilirubin encephalopathy, resulting in severe brain damage. Unfortunately, this complication still occurs despite modern medicine.

Tiny Tidbit

Eruption of discolored green primary teeth has been noted as a late complication of prolonged conjugated hyperbilirubinemia in extremely-low-birth-weight infants.

TYPES OF JAUNDICE

Physiological Jaundice

Physiological jaundice is the accumulation of bilirubin before it is changed by liver enzymes, is normal, and begins around the baby's second day of life. With a term baby, this jaundice peaks on the third or fourth day of life and then begins to decline. The bilirubin measured with this type of jaundice is known as unconjugated, indirect, or fat-soluble bilirubin (Newman, 2009).

Pathological Jaundice

Pathological jaundice is always abnormal and characterized by early onset of jaundice before 24 hours of age. The bilirubin measured with this type of jaundice is called direct or water-soluble bilirubin and can be either conjugated or unconjugated (Verklan & Walden, 2010). *Conjugated* means it is bound to liver enzymes and *unconjugated* means it is circulating loose without being bound to enzymes.

Pathological jaundice involves higher levels of bilirubin and can occur in any newborn who has an exaggerated form of physiologic jaundice or is at risk because of other factors. Risk factors for pathological jaundice include being of Asian, Native American, or East Indian descent; blood incompatibilities; excessive bruising; having a sibling treated for jaundice; viral or bacterial infection; genetic disorders; maternal gestational diabetes; maternal oxytocin (Pitocin) administration; prematurity; and metabolic disturbances such as hypoxia, acidosis, hypothermia, hypoglycemia, and starvation (Porter & Dennis, 2002; Verklan & Walden, 2010).

Breastfeeding Jaundice

Breastfeeding jaundice, also called lack of breastfeeding jaundice or starvation jaundice, is caused from lack of caloric intake, dehydration, and delayed passage of meconium in newborn infants (Porter &

Dennis, 2002). Late preterm infants are most susceptible to this exaggerated physiological jaundice because of their ineffectiveness at breastfeeding. Breastfeeding jaundice has nothing to do with the components of breast milk and everything to do with not ingesting enough breast milk; therefore, breastfeeding should not be discontinued. Instead, methods to increase effectiveness and frequency of feeding should be employed, because frequent ingestion of colostrum will help speed the passage of meconium. Supplementation may be needed until breastfeeding becomes effective and bilirubin levels decline to normal values.

Breast Milk Jaundice

Breast milk jaundice occurs after the fifth day of life, with the majority of breastfed infants either maintaining a stable but elevated bilirubin level or experiencing a second elevation in bilirubin. This level peaks around the 10th to 15th day of life (Gartner, 2001) and may continue for many weeks. Persistence of hyperbilirubinemia beyond 3 months suggests another underlying cause other than breast milk.

The mechanism of breast milk jaundice largely has been misunderstood. Hypotheses for this type of jaundice have mistakenly included:

■ Human milk contains an inhibitor of UGT, the enzyme responsible for bilirubin conjugation, and some have speculated that this blockage of conjugation causes the disorder. This hypothesis was supported by researchers who detected an unusual metabolite (progesterone, pregnane-3[α],20[β]diol) that inhibits UGT in vitro. However, not all researchers detected this unusual metabolite in breast milk or maternal urine, and the inhibitory effect of milk on the conjugating enzyme in vitro did not correlate with the timing of hyperbilirubinemia in the infants.
■ Many other hypotheses focused on the inhibition of conjugation as the likely mechanism, but suggested other inhibitors, such as increased free fatty acid concentrations resulting from excessive lipase activity in the breast milk.

The most convincing evidence of a breast milk jaundice mechanism to date (Gartner, 2001) has come from studies of the effect of breast milk on the intestinal absorption of bilirubin, resulting in increased enterohepatic circulation of bilirubin. Using a rat model, researchers found evidence that the addition of cow's milk and some human milk to the test dose of bilirubin completely inhibited intestinal absorption of bilirubin. The breast milk of mothers of infants with classical breast milk jaundice inhibited intestinal absorption for the first 2 hours, then was followed by a dramatic increase in bilirubin absorption, which continued for at least an additional 14 hours and resulted in a total absorption of 60% of the intestinal bilirubin dose. However, the factor in breast milk that increases intestinal bilirubin absorption and causes breast milk jaundice has yet to be identified.

Breast milk jaundice does not occur until after day 5 of life, apparently because the factor in breast milk that increases intestinal absorption of bilirubin is not present until after the transition from colostrum to mature milk. Gartner (2001) concludes that breast milk jaundice is neither a syndrome nor a disease, but is a normal developmental phenomenon and extension of physiological jaundice in the breastfed infant.

LATE PRETERM INFANTS HAVE INCREASED INCIDENCE AND SEVERITY OF HYPERBILIRUBINEMIA

According to several researchers, hyperbilirubinemia is one of the most common problems encountered with late preterm infants and is one of the leading causes of hospital readmissions in the late preterm infant population (Escobar et al., 2005; Hall, Simon, & Smith, 2000; Maisels & Kring, 1998; Shapiro-Mendoza et al., 2006; Tomashek et al., 2006).

Maisels and Kring (1998) examined the data from chart reviews of 29,934 infants born in a large suburban community hospital in Michigan. They compared data from those babies readmitted to hospital within 14 days of discharge with infants who were discharged during the same time frame but not readmitted to hospital. They were able to conclude that factors associated with increased risk of admission for any reason include infants of diabetic mothers, gestation less than or equal to 36 weeks, presence of jaundice before discharge, and male sex. Factors related to readmission because of jaundice were gestational age less than or equal to 36 weeks, jaundice before discharge, male sex, and breastfeeding.

WHY LATE PRETERM INFANTS ARE DISPROPORTIONATELY AFFECTED BY HYPERBILIRUBINEMIA

Increased Number of Risk Factors

The potential for hyperbilirubinemia increases as the number of risk factors for increased bilirubin increase (Porter & Dennis, 2002). Late preterm infants often experience several risk factors within the first day or two following delivery. They immediately have the risk factor of prematurity and may exhibit numerous other risk factors, such as infection, hypoxia, metabolic acidosis, hypothermia, and hypoglycemia. Many other risk factors, as listed earlier, may also be present in this population of infants.

Temperature Instability and Its Affect on Bilirubin

As discussed in Chapter 4, "Temperature Instability, Hypoglycemia, and Increased Metabolism," metabolism of brown fat, which occurs in the first few hours after birth as a mechanism of heat production, results in the release of fatty acids. These fatty acids compete with bilirubin for albumin-binding sites, resulting in increased unconjugated bilirubin levels (Mishra & Pati, 2004).

Inadequate Intake Because of Poor Breastfeeding Leading to Longer Transit Time

Breastfed newborns may be at risk for early-onset exaggerated physiologic jaundice as a result of poor feeding and inadequate intake during the first few days of life (Osborn, Reiff, & Bolus, 1984). Late preterm infants commonly demonstrate decreased volume and frequency of feedings, leading to dehydration and slower passage of meconium. The longer transit time of meconium in the intestines leads to increased enterohepatic circulation of bilirubin (Hubbard et al., 2007).

Delayed Peak in Bilirubin Levels

The total serum bilirubin (TSB) levels of term infants peaks on day 3 of life. This corresponds to approximately the time of lactogenesis II as well as time of hospital discharge. Late preterm infants' TSB usually does not peak until days 3 to 7, usually well after discharge from hospital (Verklan & Walden, 2010). Without proper follow-up and effective breastfeeding, hyperbilirubinemia quickly can ensue, and the responsibility of detecting the signs of hyperbilirubinemia is left to the ill-equipped and poorly trained parents of the late preterm infant.

ROLE OF BILIRUBIN AND KERNICTERUS: WHY LATE PRETERM INFANTS ARE MANAGED DIFFERENTLY THAN TERM INFANTS

The role of bilirubin in the development of kernicterus is poorly understood. Bhutani and Johnson (2006) studied the relationship of TSB levels, age at rehospitalization, and birth weight of infants meeting the clinical definitions of kernicterus or acute bilirubin encephalopathy and determined that these factors were similar for both late preterm and term infants, but that large-for-gestational-age and late preterm infants disproportionately developed kernicterus compared with those who were appropriate for gestational age and term.

Kernicterus is caused when unconjugated bilirubin levels exceed the binding capacity of albumin and the unbound lipid-soluble bilirubin crosses the blood–brain barrier. Albumin-bound bilirubin may also cross the blood–brain barrier if damage has occurred as a result of asphyxia, acidosis, hypoxia, hypoperfusion, hyperosmolality, or sepsis (Porter & Dennis, 2002). Late preterm infants may exhibit several of these conditions, placing them at greater risk for acute bilirubin encephalopathy.

SIMILAR SYMPTOMS, DIFFERENT MORBIDITIES

Early symptoms of bilirubin toxicity or kernicterus in newborns can include lethargy, poor feeding, high-pitched cry, and hypotonia. Late symptoms can include irritability, apnea, seizures, and fever (Porter & Dennis, 2002). All these symptoms could also be manifestations of late preterm adaptation to extra-uterine life. Lethargy, poor feeding, and hypotonia can be related to the immaturity of the infant's nervous system or to sepsis, which is common in late preterm infants. High-pitched cry, irritability, and fever can be related to sepsis or unintentional hyperthermia, such as from overdressing the infant or from overheating in a radiant warmer. Apnea can be caused from poor positioning, sepsis, central nervous system immaturity, hypothermia, or several other causes. Seizures can be caused by brain insults, sepsis, and metabolic disorders. Bilirubin and phototherapy, used to decrease bilirubin levels, both can cause excess sleepiness in an already sleepy baby.

EXTREME IMPORTANCE OF EFFECTIVE BREASTFEEDING FOR THE LATE PRETERM INFANT

Early, frequent, and effective colostrum feedings help speed the passage of meconium, thereby decreasing bilirubin levels and avoiding the consequences of hyperbilirubinemia, such as the need for phototherapy or exchange transfusion, and decreases the risk of developing kernicterus. Because of similarities in the symptoms of several morbidities, decreased thresholds for acceptable bilirubin levels, and early discharges of late preterm infants before they are proven to be breastfeeding effectively, kernicterus can be diagnosed too late, resulting in poor outcomes.

Because many factors influence the production and elimination of bilirubin, care must be taken to ensure a neutral thermal environment, decreased stimulation, decreased energy consumption, proper positioning, and adequate intake for late preterm infants. Inappropriate feeding can result in separation of mother and baby during treatment for hyperbilirubinemia and further hinders successful breastfeeding.

SIX

Unstable Respiratory Status

THE PULMONARY SYSTEM: PRESENTATION
IN LATE PRETERM INFANTS

Because the pulmonary system is one of the last systems to mature, late preterm infants are at a higher risk for respiratory distress than their full-term counterparts. They may exhibit signs of respiratory distress by grunting, flaring, retracting, becoming apneic, or being tachypneic and may need supplemental oxygen. Often the signs do not present themselves immediately and may not occur until after the baby has been placed into dyad care on the postpartum unit, with his or her parents as the primary caretakers.

EVIDENCE-BASED RESEARCH SUPPORTING
INCREASED VULNERABILITY

It is well documented that late preterm infants are much more at risk than full-term infants for respiratory distress. In a study by Wang, Doher, Fleming, and Catlin (2004), 185 newborns were identified in the electronic medical record database of Massachusetts General Hospital and were sorted into term and late preterm categories (95 and 90 infants, respectively). Chart reviews were performed to determine clinical outcomes of late preterm infants. One of the clinical outcomes that the researchers were comparing was the amount of respiratory distress encountered by each of these populations. Data showed that 26.7% of late preterm infants experienced respiratory distress compared to 4.2% of the term infants. In this study, apnea and bradycardia, although seen infrequently, were only present in the late preterm infants.

Melamed et al. (2009) determined that spontaneous late preterm deliveries carry significant neonatal morbidity, including respiratory distress. Of the infants who delivered spontaneously, 4.2% of the late preterm infants were observed with respiratory distress, compared to 0.1% of the full-term infants.

A retrospective cohort study (McIntire & Leveno, 2008) aimed at determining neonatal morbidity and mortality rates of 34-, 35-, and 36-week-gestation infants compared to term infants over a period of 18 years found that late preterm infants presented with significantly increased rates of ventilator-treated respiratory distress and transient tachypnea.

Another study (Khashu, Narayanan, Bhargava, & Osiovich, 2009) demonstrated a nearly fivefold higher occurrence of respiratory distress in late preterm infants compared to term infants.

SURFACTANT PRODUCTION AND THE STAGES OF LUNG MATURATION

Although these are just a few examples of the instability of the respiratory status of late preterm infants, it is imperative to understand the mechanism behind surfactant production, the progression of the stages of lung maturation, and other factors affecting the respiratory status of these babies. By understanding how lung maturation progresses, one is better able to appreciate the effort a late preterm infant has to put forth to adapt well to his or her extrauterine environment. A baby who is having difficulties maintaining adequate respiratory effort and oxygenation will have more difficulties with effectively breastfeeding.

Surfactant Production

Surfactant, which is a mixture of at least six phospholipids and four apoproteins, reduces surface tension in the alveoli, thereby reducing alveolar collapse at expiration (Verklan & Walden, 2010). Surfactant production begins around 24 weeks and continues to term gestation. The different admixtures peak and wane at different times throughout the fetus's lung development, and it isn't until the baby is truly term that the effective surfactant is fully and completely available. This means a late preterm infant may not have enough of the mature surfactant to maintain lung expansion, and often these babies will present well immediately after delivery, only to be admitted to the neonatal intensive care unit (NICU) or observational nursery a few hours later with respiratory distress.

Phases of Lung Development

The saccular phase of lung development occurs between 28 and 36 weeks gestation and involves the transition from sacuules, which are primitive alveoli, to alveoli, which are much more effective for gas exchange (Colin, McEvoy, & Castile, 2010). This transition is a progression, so obviously a 34- or 35-week-gestation fetus has fewer alveoli than a baby delivered at the end of 36 weeks and therefore can exhibit less effective respirations, resulting in poor gas exchange. Alveolarization, or maturation of the alveoli, occurs from 36 weeks gestation to 36 months postnatally and involves the proliferation of alveoli and progressive decrease in the size of the alveolar air spaces (Nkadi, Merritt, & Pillers, 2009). Therefore, even a baby born at 36 weeks may not have the same degree of adequate gas exchange as a full-term baby and may need some respiratory support.

COMMON PRESENTATIONS OF RESPIRATORY DISTRESS IN THE LATE PRETERM INFANT

Transient Tachypnea

Besides lack of surfactant production and lung immaturity, lack of clearance of fetal lung fluid can also cause respiratory distress in late preterm infants. Although fetal lung fluid is necessary for the proper development of the lungs, too much or too little fluid can interfere with this process. Evidence indicates that fetal lung fluid clearance is greatest as the fetus progresses toward term gestation (Helve, Pitkänen, Janér, & Andersson, 2009). If fetal lung fluid remains in the lungs after delivery, respiratory distress may ensue. Transient tachypnea of the newborn (TTN) is associated with a delay in the removal of fetal lung fluid or excessive amounts of lung fluids. Babies who are born without labor, which is often the case in emergency cesarean delivery for fetal distress or preeclampsia, both common reasons for delivery of late preterm infants, or those who are born prematurely are at risk of retaining fetal lung fluid and developing TTN (Badran et al., 2012; Derbent et al., 2011; Feldman, Woolcott, O'Connell, & Jangaard, 2012; Raju, 2012; Ramachandrappa & Jain, 2009; Verklan & Walden, 2010).

Tachypnea

Tachypnea can be caused by the late preterm infant's process of converting fat and other substrates into glucose if the infant is experiencing hypothermia or hypoglycemia (Mishra & Pati, 2004). Also, if there is inadequate nutritional intake within the first hours after birth, tachypnea can become more pronounced as the late preterm infant's body starts breaking down substrates to supply the brain with necessary glucose. This method of glucose provision requires increased oxygenation, commonly resulting in tachypnea.

Tachypnea can also be caused by hyperthermia, sepsis, and improper positioning of the late preterm infant, if positioned with his or her head flexed or extended too far sideways, causing distortion to the trachea. This is a common occurrence in late preterm infants because of hypotonia and improper positioning, whether during breastfeeding, during skin-to-skin holding, during burping, or while just holding the baby. Educating the parents to follow the correct positioning techniques as outlined in Part II of this book will help to reduce the number of infants treated for tachypnea as a result of improper positioning.

Apnea

Late preterm infants have a greater risk for apnea as a result of several underlying factors. They are more susceptible to hypoxic respiratory depression, have decreased central chemosensitivity to carbon dioxide, have immature pulmonary irritant receptors, have an increased risk for laryngeal distortion, and have decreased upper airway dilator muscle tone (Engle, Tomashek, Wallman, & Committee on the Fetus and Newborn, 2007). Improper positioning, causing distortion of the larynx, can lead to apnea and should therefore be avoided. Proper positioning techniques, as outlined in the second half of this book, should be followed to decrease the risk of apnea.

Apnea of Prematurity

Apnea of prematurity or a pause of breathing for more than 15 to 20 seconds and often accompanied by oxygen desaturation and bradycardia can occur in babies less than 37 weeks gestation. In fact, about 7% of 34- and 35-week-gestation neonates exhibit apnea of prematurity (Zhao, Gonzalez, & Mu, 2011). According to Darnall, Ariagno, and Kinney (2006), 10% of all late preterm infants have significant apnea of prematurity. Many factors may coexist or worsen apnea of prematurity, such as infection, central nervous system abnormalities, hyperthermia, glucose and electrolyte imbalances, and magnesium sulfate administration. Many of these factors are present more often in late preterm infants than they are in term infants. Altered ventilatory responses to hypoxia, hypercapnia, and altered sleep states of the late preterm infant also predispose them to this physiological immaturity of respiratory control (Zhao et al., 2011).

SEVERE RESPIRATORY DISTRESS

Because of the lung immaturity of late preterm infants, surfactant production is reduced, thereby predisposing the infant to severe respiratory distress. Hypothermia, which can result in lactic acid accumulation and metabolic acidosis, can lead to pulmonary vaso-constriction and severe respiratory distress as well (Verklan & Walden, 2010). Sepsis is also another major cause of respiratory distress in the late preterm infant population.

EFFECTS OF UNSTABLE RESPIRATORY FUNCTION ON BREASTFEEDING

Although research has definitely indicated the degree to which late preterm delivery has an effect on respiratory status, little is documented on how the late preterm's unstable respiratory status can affect breastfeeding or how breastfeeding can affect the late preterm's respiratory status.

Separation of Mother and Baby

An unstable respiratory status usually entails admission to the NICU or an observational nursery for the infant to be carefully monitored or treated. This separation of mother and baby inhibits the normal interaction, bonding, skin-to-skin contact, and on-demand feedings. Initiation of mechanical pumping and hand expression of colostrum at least every 3 hours should begin immediately upon separation of mother and baby.

Increased Metabolic Demand With Respiratory Distress

Respiratory instability leads to rapid fatigue and subsequently suboptimal breastfeeding. Babies who are experiencing breathing difficulties are usually sleepy and may be lethargic. Babies showing severe distress will be placed on NPO (nothing by mouth) status until their condition improves. Other babies who exhibit TTN or apnea of prematurity might be able to continue breastfeeding while attached to a respiratory monitor. It might prove difficult to feed a baby who is experiencing respiratory distress by breast or bottle, because he or she will not have metabolic reserves for energy consumption.

EFFECTS OF INEFFECTIVE BREASTFEEDING TECHNIQUES ON RESPIRATORY FUNCTION: LARYNGEAL DISTORTION

Poor breastfeeding technique can have a huge effect on the respiratory efforts of the late preterm infant. Laryngeal reflexes are delayed in the late preterm infant (Darnall et al., 2006), and the less rigid cartilage of the larynx can be distorted or may collapse if there is too much flexion of the head and neck. This collapse causes obstructive apnea, which is often preceded by tachypnea. Tachypnea and airway obstruction further predispose the infant to reflux and aspiration (Landry & Thompson, 2012).

Laryngeal distortion or collapse can occur during several aspects of the latching and feeding process. Direct causes of laryngeal distortion or collapse can be from placing the baby in any position that allows or requires flexion of the infant's head, such as cradle hold with the baby's head in the crook of the mother's elbow, or improper football positioning with the baby lying on his or her back and latching from under the breast. A baby placed in this type of football hold can also be suffocated by the weight of his or her mother's breast on his or her chest. While burping the baby, if the head is not supported off of the chest, laryngeal collapse can ensue. Using a baby sling before the baby is at least term gestation can also lead to laryngeal collapse and resultant respiratory distress.

Distortion of the larynx must be prevented by ensuring that the baby's chin is at a 90-degree angle with his or her chest or slightly extended and that the baby is directly facing the breast during the latch and throughout the feeding. Overextension of the neck can result in laryngeal distortion as well.

SUMMARY

Compared to full-term babies, late preterm infants are at greater risk for respiratory distress and complications from decreased oxygenation. These babies have had less time in utero, resulting in less lung maturity, less surfactant production, and less fetal lung fluid clearance. Because respiratory complications can develop later than in younger preterm infants, late preterm infants are often being cared for on the regular postpartum unit when the signs and symptoms of respiratory distress emerge. Respiratory distress is an emergency and usually results in separation of mother and baby.

Respiratory distress can lead to fatigue and suboptimal breastfeeding, and suboptimal breastfeeding techniques can lead to ineffective respiratory efforts and respiratory distress. Parents must be taught to look for signs of respiratory distress and to inform their health care professional immediately if any signs of distress are present. In addition, parents must be taught techniques for avoiding unnecessary causes of respiratory distress and understand that their late preterm infant is at a much greater risk for respiratory distress. By learning proper breastfeeding techniques, such as proper positioning and skin-to-skin contact, mothers of late preterm infants will less likely cause inadvertent respiratory insufficiency.

SEVEN

Increased Risk for Infection

IMMATURE IMMUNE SYSTEM VERSUS INCREASED EXPOSURE

It is unknown whether late preterm infants are at a higher risk of infection because of an immature immune system, or whether the increased risk stems from maternal infections that predispose these infants to preterm deliveries. Little research has been done in the area of immunity and late preterm infants.

Monocytes are important in the defense against fungal and bacterial infections (Verklan & Walden, 2010). Circulating monocytes first appear in fetal blood at about 18 weeks gestation, and by 30 weeks gestation the monocytes have increased to 3% to 7% of circulating formed blood cells (Clapp, 2006). At term birth, circulating monocyte concentrations exceed levels normally found in adults. The fact that monocyte concentrations increase with increasing gestational age may be the basis for the increased incidence of sepsis in late preterm infants compared with term infants.

Strunk et al. (2012) found that monocyte activation pathways mature as the fetus progresses to term, subjecting preterm infants to increased sepsis, especially to *Staphylococcus epidermidis.*

INCIDENCE OF INFECTION AMONG THE LATE PRETERM POPULATION

Wang, Dorer, Fleming, and Catlin (2004) randomly selected records of 120 late preterm infants born between October 1997 and October 2000 at Massachusetts General Hospital, a tertiary teaching hospital with more than 3,200 births per year. They compared these records with the records of 125 full-term infants from the same hospital and time. Late preterm infants underwent sepsis evaluations three times more frequently than full-term infants (36.7% vs. 12.6%), and although there were no significant differences as to the approach used to assess and treat suspected sepsis, more late preterm infants (30% of all evaluated late preterm infants) received 7-day antibiotic courses than full-term infants. None of the late preterm infants or term infants actually had a positive blood culture, but pneumonia was the most common diagnosis in the late preterm population.

In another study, researchers (Khashu, Narayanan, Bhargava, & Osiovich, 2009) used a population-based cohort study to examine morbidity and mortality among late preterm infants. Using data from the British Columbia Perinatal Database Registry in British Columbia, Canada, Khashu et al. analyzed all singleton births between 33 and 40 weeks gestation from April 1999 to March 2002. They compared 6,381 infants whose gestational ages were between 33 and 36 weeks with 88,867 infants who were 37 to 40 weeks gestation. Sepsis was significantly predominant in the late preterm infants (5.2 times more common). The most important associations when comparing the maternal risk factors between the two groups were the increased prevalence of chorioamnionitis and premature rupture of membranes in the late preterm group.

Tomashek et al. (2006) studied data from 1,004 late preterm infants and 24,320 term infants and concluded that late preterm infants were 1.8 times more likely to be readmitted to hospital after discharge than were term infants, with jaundice and infection accounting for the majority (77%) of readmissions.

Tsai et al. (2012) evaluated 1,491 preterm infants and 6,507 term infants in a retrospective cohort study in Taiwan. Their data showed an increased risk (3.5 times greater) for culture-proven sepsis in the late preterm infant than in the term infant.

In an observational cohort study, Cohen-Wolkowiez et al. (2009) examined 119,130 late preterm infants at 3 days old or younger and 106,142 late preterm infants between 4 days and 120 days old to determine the incidence of early-onset (during first 3 days of life) and late-onset sepsis (between days 4 and 120) in the late preterm population. The infants were admitted to 248 neonatal intensive care units (NICUs) managed by the Pediatrix Medical Group across the United States between 1996 and 2007.

Early-onset sepsis risk factors included Hispanic ethnicity, birth weight between 2,500 and 3,499 grams (5 lb, 8 oz and 7 lb, 11 oz, respectively), and cesarean delivery. The most common cause of early-onset sepsis was caused by gram-positive organisms (66.4%), followed by gram-negative organisms (27.3%), and yeast (0.8%). Approximately 29% of the infants were exposed to intrapartum antibiotics.

Late-onset sepsis risk was increased in late preterm infants born to mothers ages 11 to 19 years compared with those born to mothers ages 20 to 29 years, and late-onset sepsis was more common in late preterm infants with 5-minute Apgar scores of 0 to 3 and 4 to 6 compared to those with 5-minute Apgars higher than 6. The majority of late-onset sepsis was caused by gram-positive organisms (59.4%), followed by gram-negative organisms (30.7%) and yeast (7.7%). The most common pathogens in late-onset sepsis were *Staphylococcus aureus* and *Escherichia coli*.

WHY LATE PRETERM INFANTS EXHIBIT SIGNS OF SEPSIS

Late preterm infants commonly exhibit signs of sepsis even when sepsis is not present, which may be due to the fact that their neurological, metabolic, and respiratory systems are immature. Hubbard, Stellwagen, and Wolf (2007) sum it up by stating that late preterm infants are more frequently screened and treated for sepsis because they display possible signs of sepsis as a result of their systemic vulnerabilities, such as respiratory distress, hypoglycemia, lethargy, hypotonia, poor feeding, temperature instability, and jaundice. All of these possible signs of infection could be attributed to other aspects of late preterm infant physiology.

EFFECTIVE BREASTFEEDING TO AVOID UNNECESSARY WORKUPS FOR SEPSIS

When caring for a late preterm infant, every effort must be taken to decrease the incidences of hypoglycemia, hypothermia, respiratory distress, poor feeding, and jaundice, not only to eliminate the negative consequences of each of these morbidities but to avoid the added cost to the health care system, pain for the neonate, and stress on the parents when the infant has to experience a workup for sepsis. The infant may require admission to the NICU or special care nursery for antibiotics while sepsis is ruled out, further inhibiting breastfeeding success. With effective and timely breastfeeding, following the techniques described in Part II of this book, caregivers can decrease the chance that late preterm infants exhibit signs of sepsis when no sepsis is present and increase the early intake of colostrum, which contains many immunological properties.

EIGHT

Maternal Conditions Affecting Breast Milk Supply

COMBINATION OF WEAK SUCK, SHORT SUCKLING BURSTS, AND MATERNAL CONDITIONS ON MILK SUPPLY

Late preterm infants often cannot suckle at the breast strongly enough or long enough to stimulate the mother's nipples to bring in a full milk supply. Add to this any of the maternal conditions listed in this chapter, and the risk for a low maternal milk supply and substantial infant weight loss greatly increases. Because of this, the mothers of late preterm infants are strongly encouraged to pump their breasts for added stimulation until the baby is closer to full term and has proven to be effective at breastfeeding and the mother has a proven breast milk supply.

INSUFFICIENT MILK SUPPLY

There are many causes of delayed milk supply or insufficient milk supply stemming from maternal conditions. This decreased supply or delay in lactogenesis II (the onset of copious amounts of breast milk, or milk "coming in") can be caused from underdevelopment of breast tissue (hypoplasia), damage to the breast from surgery or injury, hormonal influences, metabolic disturbances, and medical management during pregnancy, labor, and delivery.

UNDERDEVELOPED BREASTS

Breast Hypoplasia

Breast size is generally not associated with milk-producing capabilities. However, breasts that are significantly asymmetrical or tubular or cone-shaped may be at a higher risk for producing an insufficient milk supply. Breast hypoplasia may be caused by exposure to toxic chemicals in the environment while in utero or prepuberty (Fenton, 2006), from the condition known as pectus excavatum (Park, Gu, Jang, Dhong, & Yoon, 2013), or from other factors. Hypoplastic breasts can be lacking in breast tissue on any quadrant of the breast; often the nipple and areola appear extremely large compared with the breast, and there may be a large spacing between the breasts. Breast hypoplasia is usually bilateral but can occur on one side only. Often mothers with hypoplastic breasts do not notice a change in size or shape of the breasts during pregnancy, although many will have an enlargement and darkening of the areola. Because of the hypoplasia, milk-producing tissue of the breast may be insufficient or may be completely lacking. Especially with a late preterm infant, do not assume that the hypoplastic breast can produce a full supply of milk, and if the baby shows any signs of inadequate intake despite appropriate breastfeeding, supplementation should be begun immediately. Encourage frequent, unlimited breastfeeding; pumping and hand expression; and rental or purchase of a multiuser, hospital-grade pump until milk supply is fully established or it becomes evident that the milk supply is insufficient. This is a difficult subject to discuss with a mother, but she needs to be aware of the possible limitations, as well as the steps she can do to increase her chances for a full or partial breast milk supply. A lactation consultant may be able to discuss this delicate matter most appropriately.

BREAST SURGERY OR INJURY TO THE BREAST

Breast Surgery or Nipple Piercing

Any breast surgery or injury can interrupt the normal tissue integrity and create scar tissue, which may block the flow of breast milk. The more menstrual periods the woman has after the surgery, the higher the likelihood of nerve innervations and tissue repair to the breast, reversing this damage.

Nipple piercing can cause scar tissue formation, blocking the flow of breast milk while increasing engorgement along the tract behind the scar tissue. Usually only one section of the breast is affected. Breast massage and compressions may assist in increasing the milk flow, but often that area of breast tissue initially becomes engorged, then stops producing breast milk because of lack of breast milk removal. Ice packs after feeding or pumping can help alleviate pain and discomfort associated with the engorgement.

Breast Augmentation

Breast augmentation falls under the category of breast surgery but can cause some other issues with milk supply as well. It is important to ascertain whether the mother had hypoplastic breasts or a large gap between the breasts before the surgery. Also important is whether or not the mother has sensation in the areola and nipple, because lack of sensation can be associated with nerve damage and decreased nipple stimulation, leading to a decreased spike in prolactin levels and decreased milk supply. Lack of sensation also predisposes the mother to increased risk for nipple damage, because she may not be aware of an improperly latched baby and significant damage can be done if she is unaware of the poor latch.

The surgery itself can disrupt the flow of breast milk, especially if the nipple has been removed during the procedure. Scarring from excision around the entire areola is much more concerning than scarring below the areola or below the breast. Hurst (1996) compared lactation sufficiency between augmented women and nonaugmented women and found that among 42 augmented women, 27 (64%) has insufficient lactation. Among the 42 nonaugmented women in the study, only three women (less than 7%) had insufficient supply. Also noted was the type of breast incision affecting supply. Hurst noted that the periareolar approach was far more likely to decrease lactation outcomes compared with the submammary-axillary approach.

Another concern is the type of filler used in the augmentation process. Wang et al. (2012) describe polyacrylamide hydrogel (PAAG) as a widely used substance in augmentations performed in Russia, China, and Iran. However, like other fillers used previously in the United States, there is a high incidence of breast infection reported during breastfeeding (greater than 50% infection rate), resulting in the surgical removal of galactoceles or intraprosthetic collection of sterile pus. Some of the materials used before silicone implants caused leakage and adhesions of the breast, leading to distortion of the breast, calcifications, hypertrophy, and decreased milk supply.

Andrade, Coca, and Abrão (2010) compared women with breast reductions, women with augmentations, and women without breast procedures to compare breastfeeding patterns. Their results showed the probability of an infant being exclusively breastfed at the end of the first month was 80% in women without surgery, 54% in women with augmentation, and 29% in women with reduction surgery. Among women with breast augmentation surgery, the risk of an infant being nonexclusively breastfeeding at 1 month was 2.6 times greater than that of the infant of the mother without breast surgery.

Breast Reduction and Breast Lift

The usual technique for breast reduction is the transposition technique in which the nipple-areola complex remains attached to the breast gland on a pedicle (a flap or stalk) and an underside wedge of the breast is removed from the sides. The ability to breast-feed after this surgery depends on the integrity of the milk ducts, nerve pathways, and blood supply, as well as on the amount of glandular tissue removed. Research from Brazil (Souto, Giugliani, Giugliani, & Schneider, 2003) resulted in significantly decreased exclusive breastfeeding at both 1-month and 4-month marks. At 1 month, 70% of women without breast reduction surgery were exclusively breastfeeding compared with 21% of the breast reduction mothers. At 4 months, these rates decreased to 22% in women without the surgery and only 4% in those women who had the breast reduction surgery.

Breast lifts involve one of three different incisions. A donut incision is made around the border of the areola; a keyhole or lollipop incision involves incisions around the areola and extending vertically from the areola to the breast crease; and the most common incision is the anchor incision, which resembles the keyhole with additional incisions made along each breast crease. The surgeon then manipulates the breast tissue to a higher area, repositions the nipple, and sutures are placed deep in the breast tissue to hold the breast up. Excess skin is cut off. Additionally, large areolas are trimmed to size.

Both breast reduction surgery and breast lifts interrupt the integrity of the breast tissue, leaving a large risk of insufficient milk supply. In addition, there is an increased possibility of not having a connection from the milk ducts through to the nipple tip for breast milk to be removed.

HORMONAL CAUSES OF INSUFFICIENT MILK SUPPLY

Hormonal conditions such as polycystic ovarian syndrome (PCOS), thyroid abnormalities, and Sheehan's syndrome can all negatively affect maternal milk supply.

Polycystic Ovarian Syndrome

Although the complex syndrome known as PCOS is not fully understood, it is considered to be a syndrome of ovarian, endocrine, and metabolic dysfunction and is associated with infertility, cardiovascular disease, and diabetes. The hormonal abnormalities that occur with PCOS are associated with milk supply issues (Marasco, Marmet, & Shell, 2000). Although some mothers with minimal hormonal abnormalities may produce an abundant supply of breast milk, others who present with hypothyroidism, obesity, insulin resistance, and altered estrogen may experience a much more diminished supply. PCOS can also result in increased rates of preeclampsia, gestational diabetes, and premature deliveries.

Hypothyroidism

Thyroid glands control metabolism; they are involved with the hormones of pregnancy and lactation and are necessary for normal breast development and initiation of lactation. Low thyroid levels have been associated with low milk supply, although the best research available is on rat, mice, and bovine models (Lisboa et al., 2010). Data from a study on mice indicated that thyroid hormones are necessary for a galactopoietic (milk-producing) response to growth hormone and prolactin (Capuco, Kahl, Jack, Bishop, & Wallace, 1999); without the necessary thyroid hormones, the baby mice did not gain weight. Hapon, Simoncini, Via, and Jahn (2003) demonstrated that hypothyroidism can decrease serum oxytocin concentrations, decreasing the milk ejection reflex and leading to excess weight loss in baby rats.

Uncontrolled hypothyroidism in pregnancy can lead to preterm birth, low birth weight, and mental retardation (Drews & Seremak-Mrozikiewicz, 2011).

Hyperthyroidism

Some women experience an abundance of breast milk production while in a hyperthyroid state, but others have a low milk ejection reflex, leading to lactation failure. Hyperthyroidism in rats is associated with early onset of lactogenesis II (milk "coming in"), but impaired release of oxytocin for milk ejection leads to a lower volume of milk released at ejection, lower weight gain in the infants, and early mammary involution and cessation of milk production (Varas et al., 2002). Hyperthyroidism also changes maternal liver and mammary lipid metabolism. A study by Varas, Jahn, and Giménez (2001) demonstrated decreased lipid concentrations, despite increased rate of synthesis in the liver, and decreased mammary synthesis of lipids, leading to a decreased rate of growth in the babies of hyperthyroid mothers.

Sheehan's Syndrome

Sheehan's syndrome is a rare complication of pregnancy, usually occurring after excessive blood loss, as with postpartum hemorrhage or abruption (Kilicli, Dokmetas, & Acibucu, 2013). Major hemorrhage or hypotension during the peripartum period can result in ischemia of the anterior pituitary, leading to necrosis of that region. The most common initial symptoms of Sheehan's syndrome are difficulties with or absence of lactation. Occasionally, the diagnosis is not made until years later when there are further features of hypopituitarism.

Retained Placental Fragments

Although little is written about the effect of retained placental fragments on lactation, we know that the expulsion of the placenta decreases progesterone levels and subsequently increases the release of prolactin, which is necessary for lactogenesis II (Forsling et al., 1979; Neville & Morton, 2001). Without complete placenta expulsion, progesterone levels may remain elevated, interfering with prolactin release and therefore inhibiting the onset of lactogenesis II.

Theca Lutein Cyst

Though uncommon, theca lutein cysts, which cause the ovaries to be enlarged by multiple cysts during pregnancy, create a delay in lactogenesis II because the cysts produce a high level of testosterone, which suppresses milk production. It can take up to 4 weeks or more after delivery for the testosterone levels to fall enough to initiate the milk supply (Betzold, Hoover, & Snyder, 2004; Hoover, Barbalinardo, & Platia, 2002).

METABOLIC CAUSES OF IMPAIRED MILK SUPPLY

Diabetes

A delay in the onset of lactogenesis II is often exhibited in women with poorly controlled diabetes (Arthur, Smith, & Hartmann, 1989). In women with insulin-dependent diabetes mellitus, lactogenesis II generally takes an additional 24 hours to attain the concentrations of nondiabetic women, as measured by the markers of lactose, citrate, and total nitrogen (Hartmann & Cregan, 2001). Oliveira, Cunha, Penha-Silva, Abdallah, and Jorge (2008) evaluated the interference of type 1 diabetes mellitus with the onset of lactogenesis II and found that women with inadequate glycemic control had an 18-hour delay to achieve lactogenesis II compared to women without diabetes, and that there was a significantly lower lactose concentration of breast milk in the diabetic women in the third and fifth days postpartum compared with the women without diabetes, signifying a decreased breast milk supply.

Obesity

Several studies have addressed the fact that mothers who are overweight or obese (body mass index greater than 26) are less likely to initiate breastfeeding, have a delay in onset of lactogenesis II, and are inclined to have earlier cessation of breastfeeding than women who are not overweight. Rasmussen and Kjolhede (2004) examined the effects of obesity on the prolactin response to infant suckling, assuming progesterone was the factor that caused a delay in milk production. However, they found that not to be the case. Instead, after making adjustments for confounding factors, they found overweight/obesity as the only significant negative predictor of prolactin response.

Lap Banding and Bariatric Surgery

Often women undergo weight reduction surgery in an effort to lose weight. It is unknown if breastfeeding failure as a result of bariatric (weight loss) surgery is due to the effects of the surgery or to the fact that obese women have bariatric surgery and obesity is a risk factor for decreased breastfeeding success. If the reason for the obesity is because of hormones, the surgery does not affect these hormones and the same hormones that were causing the weight gain can still interfere with lactogenesis II. Weight reduction surgeries are classified as restrictive, malabsorptive, or a combination of the two, so the other concern with weight loss surgery is the need for appropriate caloric intake and absorption of all necessary nutrients. Because the mother can only ingest small amounts of food at a time, it is important that she makes smart decisions about the nutritional content of her meals and that she consumes enough calories to sustain lactation. In healthy women, the Institute of Medicine (1991) recommends no more than a 4-pound weight loss per month while lactating. Adequate levels of maternal vitamin B_{12}, as well as levels of all other nutrients, should be maintained within normal ranges. Inadequate levels of maternal vitamin B_{12} can result in infants with failure to thrive, anemia, hypotonia, poor feeding, and severe neurological damage (National Institutes of Health, 2011).

Maternal Anemia

Maternal anemia may be caused from insufficient iron intake, blood loss, or other factors. Henly et al. (1995) explored the relationship between anemia and insufficient breast milk supply in 630 primiparous women and identified anemia as associated with the development of an insufficient milk supply, which resulted in early cessation of breastfeeding.

Postpartum Hemorrhage

Postpartum hemorrhage is associated with hypovolemia, anemia, and increased breast milk sodium levels and can possibly lead to Sheehan's syndrome (discussed earlier). Willis and Livingstone (1995) examined the association of insufficient milk syndrome in causing failure to thrive in infants with maternal postpartum hemorrhage. Several of the failure-to-thrive infants suffered hypernatremic dehydration, presumably from the high mammary sodium levels.

MEDICAL MANAGEMENT CAUSES OF IMPAIRED MILK SUPPLY

In a study examining the incidence and risk factors for suboptimal infant breastfeeding behavior, delayed onset of lactation, and excess neonatal weight loss among mother–infant pairs in a population of highly educated and highly motivated women, Dewey, Nommsen-Rivers, Heinig, and Cohen (2003) determined that there are several factors that significantly and negatively affect breastfeeding. Factors that influenced suboptimal infant breastfeeding behavior included cesarean section, stage II labor longer than 1 hour, and birth weight less than 3,600 grams (7 lb, 14.9 oz), among other things. Delayed onset of lactation (greater than 72 hours) was associated with primiparity, cesarean section, stage II labor longer than 1 hour, flat or inverted nipples, and other factors. Excess weight loss in infants was associated with primiparity, long duration of labor, use of labor medications in multiparas, and other factors. The risk of excess infant weight loss was 7.1 times greater if the mother had delayed onset of lactogenesis II and 2.6 times greater if the infant exhibited suboptimal feeding behaviors during the first 24 hours after birth.

Pitocin Induction

Administration of synthetic oxytocin (pitocin) has been associated with delayed initiation of breastfeeding (Wiklund, Norman, Uvnäs-Moberg, Ransjö-Arvidson, & Andolf, 2009) and interference with the release of endogenous oxytocin. Bell, White-Traut, and Rankin (2012) demonstrated through videos of infants 45 to 50 minutes after birth that infants exposed to intrapartum synthetic oxytocin were 11.5 times likely to show low to medium levels of prefeeding organization compared to high levels of prefeeding organization demonstrated by unexposed infants.

Epidural Analgesia

Wiklund et al. (2009) examined early breastfeeding behaviors in full-term newborns whose mothers had received epidural analgesia during an uncomplicated labor and compared them to similar infants of mothers who had not received epidurals. Their findings indicate that significantly fewer babies whose mothers received epidurals suckled at the breast within 4 hours of life, were more often given artificial milk during their hospital stay, and fewer were fully breastfeeding at discharge.

Gizzo et al. (2012) found that when comparing labor with epidurals against labor without epidurals, among neonatal parameters the only statistical difference was for the timing of the first feeding, with a mean duration of less than 30 minutes in 62% of nonepidural dyads versus only 29% of the epidural dyads.

In a study involving 772 breastfeeding dyads within the first 30 days postpartum, after adjusting for standard demographics and intrapartum factors, Dozier et al. (2013) found that epidural anesthesia significantly predicted breastfeeding cessation.

Cesarean Section

Mathur et al. (1993) found that women who had undergone elective cesareans and received spinal anesthesia were much more likely to initiate early breastfeeding than those who had undergone an emergency cesarean and received general anesthesia. Sakalidis et al. (2013) found that babies who had been delivered by cesarean and whose mothers used pethidine (meperidine) patient-controlled epidural analgesia (PCEA) after delivery showed faster suckling rates, later times to first breastfeeding, breast fullness, and lower neurobehavioral scores than those infants born vaginally. Woods et al. (2012) assessed patient-controlled epidural analgesia (PCEA) versus patient-controlled analgesia (PCA) after cesarean delivery and concluded that PCEA confers greater pain control than PCA and that women with greater pain control are more likely to breastfeed six or more times in the first 24 hours after delivery.

Dewey et al. (2003) determined cesarean section to be significantly associated with suboptimal infant breastfeeding behavior, delayed onset of lactogenesis II, and excess infant weight loss when labor medications used, as is the case with cesareans. Hellmeyer et al. (2012) examined outcomes of 893 late preterm infants for several factors and found that late preterm infants born by cesarean section were at a significantly higher risk of developing hypoglycemia than those born by vaginal delivery.

Intrapartum Intravenous Fluid Administration

To determine the effect of conservative versus usual intrapartum intravenous (IV) fluid management in low-risk women receiving epidural analgesia on weight loss in breastfed newborns, Watson, Hodnett, Armson, Davies, and Watt-Watson (2012) randomly assigned women into either a conservative care group or the usual care group. Two hundred women participated, with 100 women in each group. Forty-eight infants in the usual care group and 44 infants in the restricted fluid group lost greater than 7% of their birth weight before discharge. The researchers conclude that restriction of IV fluids does not affect newborn weight when volumes of IV fluid are less than 2,500 mLs, but exploratory analyses suggest that breastfed newborn weight loss increases when intrapartum volumes greater than 2,500 mLs are infused.

Excess intrapartum IV fluid administration may also lead to fluid overload, causing engorgement of the nipple, areola, and breast tissue, which results in latch difficulties and subsequent decreased breast milk intake by the infant.

OTHER FACTORS AFFECTING BREAST MILK SUPPLY

Twins and triplets are another reason for insufficient milk supply. Although patience and vigilance to proper nipple stimulation and milk removal should pay off in long-term milk production, short-term effects may be exhibited because there is not enough colostrum or breast milk to go around.

Tiny Tidbit

Alcohol is not a galactagogue, as some may believe. It decreases the magnitude and frequency of the milk ejection reflex, thereby decreasing breast emptying, which can lead to insufficient milk supply.

Another concern is the situation where the mother's nipples are too big for a late preterm baby to effectively latch. If the baby just latches to the nipple, very little milk transfer is likely to occur, nipple pain can ensue, and lack of breast emptying and stimulation lead to further lactation decline.

Tiny Tidbit

A family history of alcoholism can be associated with decreased prolactin response.

SUMMARY

Many conditions affecting pregnant women and the course of their labor and delivery can interfere with the normal lactation process and the initiation of a sufficient milk supply. A mother who is already having a delay in milk production will likely have an even longer delay or insufficient supply if attempting to breastfeed a late preterm infant without assistance. If we fail to properly educate the mother on the cause of the delay of milk initiation, the complications of breastfeeding late preterm infants, and the necessary steps involved in obtaining a full milk supply and successful breastfeeding, it is highly likely that mother will become frustrated and helpless and early cessation of breastfeeding will ensue.

NINE

Maternal Self-Esteem and Its Effect on Breastfeeding

FACTORS ASSOCIATED WITH LOW MATERNAL SELF-ESTEEM

Women with low self-esteem are much less likely to initiate breastfeeding than other women. Often women with low self-esteem are overweight or obese, adolescent, low income, or from a culture where social discrimination begins at birth. A woman who has low self-esteem will likely find breastfeeding a late preterm infant very intimidating, both mentally and physically, as she now takes on the role of sole provider of infant nutrition.

LOW SELF-ESTEEM AND THE PERCEPTION OF LOW SUPPLY

Researchers have found that the perception of insufficient milk supply is a major indicator of breastfeeding non-initiation or early cessation. McCarter-Spaulding and Kearney (2001) used a cross-sectional descriptive correlation study of 60 breastfeeding dyads, with infants 1 to 11 weeks old, from four primary care pediatric practices in the northern United States. Using the Perception of Insufficient Milk questionnaire, the investigators found a significant correlation between self-efficacy (the measure of one's own ability to complete tasks and reach goals) and perceived insufficient milk scores.

Using a prospective cohort study, Mehta, Siega-Riz, Herring, Adair, and Bentley (2011) examined the correlation between overweight or obesity, psychological factors during pregnancy, and breastfeeding initiation. Women who began pregnancy overweight or obese (body mass index [BMI] equal to or greater than 26) had almost four times the risk of not initiating breastfeeding compared to underweight or normal weight women. In this study, depressive symptoms, perceived stress, anxiety, and self-esteem levels during pregnancy were not associated with pregravid BMI and breastfeeding initiation.

Another study, done in Brisbane, Australia (Blyth et al., 2002) examined 300 women in the last trimester of pregnancy and again at 1 week and 4 months postpartum to assess infant feeding methods and breastfeeding confidence using the Breastfeeding Self-Efficacy Scale. Although 92% of the women initiated breastfeeding, by 4 months only 28.6% were exclusively breastfeeding and 40% had discontinued breastfeeding altogether. Antenatal and 1-week Breastfeeding Self-Efficacy Scale scores were significantly related to breastfeeding outcomes at 1 week and 4 months.

A self-administered, closed-ended questionnaire was introduced to 694 low-income women who were certified for Women, Infants, and Children (WIC, a U.S. food and nutrition program for low-income women and children younger than age 5) in Mississippi (Mitra, Khoury, Hinton, & Carothers, 2004). Women who intended to breast-feed had higher levels of breastfeeding knowledge and self-efficacy and reported fewer barriers to breastfeeding than those not intending to breastfeed. Perceived social support was included as an independent predictor of breastfeeding intention.

O'Brian, Buikstra, Fallon, and Hegney (2009) analyzed their research and identified 45 psychological factors thought to influence the duration of breastfeeding. Factors that were considered most important included the mother's priorities, mothering self-efficacy, faith in breast milk, adaptability, stress, and breastfeeding self-efficacy.

Analyzing data from 159 mothers who delivered their infants in a large Queensland maternity hospital during 1997, researchers (Papinczak & Turner, 2000) aimed to determine the degree to which certain personal and social maternal factors in the immediate postpartum period and the next 6 months were associated with the length of breastfeeding duration. The study found that longer breastfeeding duration was most significantly associated with increased breastfeeding self-confidence, lower levels of anxiety and depression, increased self-esteem and coping capacity, and stronger social health.

Laufer (1990) makes a great point, saying that how the birth process is managed may have a huge impact on breastfeeding success. What may appear to health care professionals as a routine delivery may be perceived by the mother as humiliating or dehumanizing. If the mother has an extremely negative perception of her birth experience, she may suffer a loss of self-esteem, preferring not to breastfeed as a way to salvage her dignity amid the uncertainty of breastfeeding success or perceived failure.

Finally, Padovani, Duarte, Martinez, and Linhares (2011) assessed a sample of 50 mothers of preterm infants and 25 mothers of full-term infants using State-Trait Anxiety Inventory and Beck Depression Inventory, focusing on breastfeeding issues. The mothers of the preterm infants reported more uncertainties and worries about breastfeeding and identified more obstacles for successful breastfeeding than the mothers of the full-term infants. Maternal reports were associated directly with the neonate's clinical status: Lower birth weight, higher clinical risk, and longer hospital stay increased mothers' worries and perceived obstacles.

PERCEPTION OF LOW SUPPLY AND ITS EFFECT ON BREASTFEEDING SUCCESS: WHAT MEDICAL PROFESSIONALS CAN DO TO DEBUNK THIS MYTH

Because we know self-esteem plays a large part in breastfeeding failure or success, with a strong influence on perceived breast milk supply, we have our work cut out for us as medical professionals. Proper education about colostrum production, method of delivery, the length of time that breast milk supply typically takes to increase greatly, and normal infant stomach capacity should be initiated before delivery. A great time for practitioners to begin this teaching is around 16 to 18 weeks gestation, when colostrum production begins. Teaching the mother about the benefits of early colostrum feedings, assuring her that appropriate assistance will be available, and encouraging her to believe in herself will benefit greatly. Take the time to discuss any concerns the mother may have at this point.

As the mother and fetus approach late preterm gestation, if there is any indication of possible late preterm delivery, practitioners should discuss not only the respiratory status of this gestation, but reasonable breastfeeding expectations and late preterm infant complications. If at all possible, this should be done in a relaxed atmosphere, not under the stress of an imminent delivery. If a mother knows what to expect, she has time to rationalize and process the information, leading to less disappointment and better self-efficacy. Again, take the time to discuss any concerns the mother might have about giving birth to a late preterm infant and about breastfeeding that late preterm infant. If appropriate, refer the mother to an experienced lactation consultant who can further educate the mother before delivery.

Refrain from stating that as long as the baby is breathing well, he or she will be fine. We know there are other real potential complications and we shouldn't give the parents a false sense of security. Instead, state that one of the major complications of late preterm infants is lung immaturity, and once the baby overcomes that, the other hurdles will be smaller.

Postpartum nurses and pediatricians should continue this discussion of late preterm vulnerability with the parents, ensuring appropriate, timely, and nonconflicting information and assistance.

SUMMARY

A mother who is well educated about late preterm infants will have a much easier time adapting to the challenges that her late preterm infant will face. Education increases self-esteem and self-efficacy of breastfeeding, which leads to increased empowerment. Knowing ahead of time that the baby will require at least some assistance with breastfeeding will take away some of the mother's self-blame, indicating that it is the baby who is not fully capable of breastfeeding and not the mother who is incapable of breastfeeding. Unanticipated problems can negatively affect breastfeeding outcomes even of those who have great intentions of exclusively breastfeeding. Working together, medical professionals can increase mothers' self-confidence and influence a better breastfeeding outcome for late preterm infants.

TEN

The Risks of Not Breastfeeding

WHY BREASTFEED?

Many people might ask, *Why breastfeed if it is so difficult, especially with a late preterm infant?* The answer is simply because in most cases, breastfeeding is best for both the baby and the mother. Breastfeeding is considered to be the gold standard for newborn and infant feeding, and any other form of feeding should be considered a less optimal substitute.

It has been well documented that breastfeeding, compared to formula feeding, is best for many reasons. Breastfeeding far outweighs the risks of formula feeding in babies of any gestation and is also beneficial for the mother's well-being. Add to that the cost of formula and the carbon footprint bottle feeding leaves behind, and the real question is, *Why wouldn't you breastfeed?*

Tiny Tidbit

Jury duty can be postponed for up to 12 months for breastfeeding mothers.

RISKS OF NOT BREASTFEEDING THE LATE PRETERM INFANT

Impaired Neurological Functioning

Recent research has shown that late preterm infants often face increased impaired neurological and developmental outcomes compared to full-term infants. There may be persistent developmental and cognitive concerns, as well as increased need for special education through at least fifth grade, for babies born late preterm (Odd, Emond, & Whitelaw, 2012; Lipkind, Slopen, Pfeiffer, & McVeigh, 2012). Late preterm infants may have lower reading and math scores (Lipkind et al., 2012) than their full-term counterparts and be at a 36% higher risk for developmental delays (Morse, Zheng, Tang, & Roth, 2009). Breastfeeding helps boost protection from further neurological decline, which is especially important for late preterm infants, who are already at a disadvantage.

Although widely researched over the past several decades, the relationship of breastfeeding to cognitive development has been elusive. Whereas experts agree that children who are breastfed are generally more intelligent, it is unclear whether this advantage is due to the effects of breastfeeding or other accompanying characteristics of women who breastfeed.

Daniels and Adair (2005) attempted a new approach to the theory that breastfeeding makes babies smarter. They evaluated the relationship between breastfeeding and cognitive development in a population in whom breastfeeding was inversely correlated with socioeconomic advantages and other healthy maternal behaviors. The researchers studied 1,790 normal-birth-weight infants and 189 low-birth-weight (< 2500 g) infants in metropolitan Cebu, Philippines, and followed them from birth through middle childhood. Cognitive ability was assessed using the Philippines Nonverbal Intelligence Test at the ages of 8.5 and again at 11.5 years. After controlling for confounding variables, scores at 8.5 years were higher for infants who were breastfed longer (12 to less than 18 months vs. less than 6 months). Although still positive, results at age 11.5 years were slightly less impressive. This investigation highlights the importance of long-term breastfeeding even after the introduction of complementary foods.

Even if people dispute the fact that breastfeeding can make you smarter, research proves that smarter women breastfeed!

Increased Risk for Infection

Breastfeeding increases the amount of immunoglobulins the baby receives, helping to boost the immune responses of the baby when subjected to pathogens. Colostrum and breast milk help close the gaps in the gut lining, protecting the infant from added irritation and infection of the gut. Because a late preterm infant is more susceptible to infection, breastfeeding is a very important protective action a mother can take to reduce the risk for her child.

Increased Risk for Hyperbilirubinemia and Jaundice

Breastfeeding, especially the ingestion of colostrum in the first few days, helps speed up transit time in the gut, thereby decreasing exposure to bilirubin. The more colostrum the baby receives, the quicker the clearance of meconium and appropriate adaptation to normal stooling, decreasing the risk of jaundice and hyperbilirubinemia.

Increased Risk for Increased Metabolic Demands

Researchers studied the effect of breastfeeding duration of 100 preterm infants (30–36 weeks gestation) to analyze their nutritional and metabolic markers at 6 to 9 months of life (Monroy-Torres, Naves-Sánchez, & Ortega-Garcia, 2012). They compared metabolic indicators, including but not limited to hemoglobin, glucose, cholesterol, triglycerides, and insulin, and compared them with the general recommendations for this group of babies. The average duration of breastfeeding was 4.3 months. Results showed significant differences with regard to reference values in babies who had shorter breastfeeding duration. The researchers concluded that premature infants showed deficiencies in weight gain and recommended prolonging breastfeeding duration to maintain appropriate weight and nutrition.

THE REAL RISKS OF FORMULA FEEDING

Formula Feeding Risks to Infants

- More diarrhea, vomiting, and gastrointestinal infections (Aguiar & Silva, 2011; Boccolini, Boccolini, de Carvalho, & de Oliveira, 2012; Dey et al., 2013; Kramer & Kakuma, 2012; Ma, Brewer-Asling, & Magnus, 2013; Morales et al., 2012; Muñoz-Quezada et al., 2013)
- Decreased response to vaccines (Dórea, 2012)
- More ear infections (Abrahams & Labbok, 2011; Aguiar & Silva, 2011)
- Higher rates of respiratory syncytial virus (RSV) and other respiratory infections (Aguiar & Silva, 2011; Ma et al., 2013)

- Increased risk of sudden infant death syndrome (SIDS; Aguiar & Silva, 2011; Hauck, Thompson, Tanabe, Moon, & Vennemann, 2011; Ma et al., 2013)
- More allergies (Morales et al., 2012; Turck et al., 2005)
- More eczema (Morales et al., 2012)
- May decrease intelligence (as measured by IQ) by up to 8% (Horwood & Ferguson, 1998; Kramer et al., 2008; Turck et al., 2005)
- Increased risk of obesity (Koletzko et al., 2013; Sloan, Gildea, Stewart, Sneddon, & Iwaniec, 2008)
- Decreased social development and status (Martin, Goodall, Gunnell, & Davey Smith, 2007)
- Increased risk of cancer (Aguiar & Silva, 2011)
- Increased risk for juvenile diabetes (Alves, Figueiroa, Meneses, & Alves, 2012)
- More psychological, behavioral, and learning problems (Shelton, Collishaw, Rice, Harold, & Thapar, 2011)
- Increased risk of contamination during food preparation, leading to food poisoning

Formula Feeding Risks to Mothers

- Higher risk for obesity (Bobrow, Quigley, Green, Reeves, & Beral, 2012)
- Slower uterine involution and greater risk of hemorrhage (Leung, 2005)
- Increased insulin requirements for diabetic mothers (Chouinard-Castonguay, Weisnagel, Tchernof, & Robitaille, 2013)
- Increased risk of type 2 diabetes (Schwartz et al., 2009; Ziegler et al., 2012)
- Increased risk for hypertension and cardiovascular disease (Schwartz et al., 2009)
- Increased risk of breast, uterine, ovarian, and endometrial cancer (Aguiar & Silva, 2011; Jordan, Cushing-Haugen, Wicklund, Doherty, & Rossing, 2012)
- Increased osteoporosis (Turck et al., 2005)
- Decreased maternal–child bonding (Leung, 2005)
- Less convenient
- More expensive (Ma et al., 2013)

Formula Feeding Risks to the Environment

- Increased amount of pollution caused by manufacturing, packaging, and disposal

- Increased carbon footprint
- Increased cost to government agencies that supply formula to low-income families

THE FINANCIAL COST OF NOT BREASTFEEDING

Researchers set out to estimate the potential cost savings to individual states if families were to meet the current recommendations for exclusive breastfeeding for the first 6 months of life. They used Louisiana as a case study to develop the framework of their research and examined four specific infant diseases: respiratory tract infections, gastroenteritis, necrotizing enterocolitis, and SIDS. Using cost-analyses methods, cost savings and case and death reductions related to these illnesses were calculated. They determined that a total of $216,103,368 could be saved and 18 infant deaths could be prevented from just these diseases alone if 90% of newborns in Louisiana were exclusively breastfed for the first 6 months. With 80% compliance, $186,371,125 in savings could occur and 16 infant deaths could be avoided (Ma et al., 2013).

In a similar study, Bartick and Reinhold (2010) conducted a cost analysis for all pediatric diseases for which the Agency for Healthcare Research and Quality reported risk ratios that favored breastfeeding: otitis media, necrotizing enterocolitis, gastroenteritis, hospitalization for pneumonia, atopic dermatitis, asthma, leukemia, SIDS, type 1 diabetes mellitus, and childhood obesity. They used 2005 Centers for Disease Control and Prevention (CDC) breastfeeding rates and 2007 dollars and determined that if 90% of U.S. families complied with medical recommendations to exclusively breastfeed for 6 months, the United States would save $13 billion per year and prevent more than 900 deaths, most of whom would be infants. If even 80% of families complied with the recommendation, the United States would save $10.5 billion and 741 deaths would be avoided.

PROTECTION AGAINST MATERNAL BREAST AND OTHER CANCERS: A VERY COMPELLING ARGUMENT FOR BREASTFEEDING

If the evidence of the impact of breastfeeding for the baby is not enough to convince mothers to breastfeed, perhaps the following studies on the impact for the mother may be more compelling.

A multitude of research has confirmed that breastfeeding has a very significant protective mechanism to greatly decrease the risk of cancer in women who breastfeed their infants. A study by Jordan et al. (2012) used the data from 881 women who had breastfed and 1,345 women who had not breastfed. Their results showed that women who ever breastfed had a 22% reduction in risk of ovarian cancer compared with those who never breastfed, and the risk reduction appeared greater with longer durations of breastfeeding per breastfed child. The risk reduction appeared greatest for the endometrioid and clear cell subtypes.

Yanhua et al. (2012) conducted a case-control study on 263 breast cancer cases and 457 non–breast cancer controls and found significant independent positive associations between breast cancer and never breastfeeding.

In a review by Do Carmo França-Botelho, Ferreira, França, França, and Honório-França (2012), the authors conclude that rates of breast cancer are decreased in women who have a history of breastfeeding. They claim breastfeeding reduces the risk of breast cancer because of the differentiation of breast tissue and the reduction in the lifetime number of ovulation cycles. In addition, they mention alpha-lactalbumin as one of the primary components of breast milk thought to cause tumor cell death.

Msolly, Gharbi, and Ben Ahmed (2013) examined the relationship between menstrual and reproductive factors and their link to breast cancer, using a case-control study of 400 women in Tunisia. They found a significantly reduced risk of breast cancer for those women whose lifetime duration of breastfeeding was 73 to 108 months or longer.

Sugawara et al. (2013) analyzed data for 26,680 women between the ages of 40 and 79 years. During the 11-year follow-up there were 148 cases of breast cancer and 32 cases of endometrial cancer in these women. The researchers found a strong possibility that not breastfeeding is positively associated with increased risk for both breast and endometrial cancer.

Researchers collected data from 47 epidemiological studies in 30 countries to determine whether breastfeeding has a protective effect against breast cancer (Collaborative Group on Hormonal Factors in Breast Cancer, 2002). They found that the relative risk for breast cancer decreased by 4.3% for every 12 months of breastfeeding.

BREASTFEEDING AND THE RISK OF DEATH

Becher, Bhushan, and Lyon (2012) examined the population incidence of sudden and unexpected postnatal collapse of 45 infants who were at least 37 weeks gestation. All the infants had an Apgar score of at least 8 at 5 minutes but collapsed within 12 hours in hospital, required positive-pressure ventilation, and either died or received ongoing intensive care. In one third of the infants (15/45), an underlying disease or abnormality was detected. In 24 of the remaining 45 infants, the diagnosis was airway obstruction during breastfeeding or while in a prone position. The mothers were commonly primiparous and were alone with their infants when the collapse occurred. Of the 30 infants without underlying disease, 22 (73%) developed postasphyxial encephalopathy, 5 died, and 5 had neurological sequelae at 1 year of age.

Some people may interpret this research as a wakeup call to the harms of breastfeeding, so they may believe formula feeding is advantageous. That's like saying scissors can cut you, so we are banning all scissors. If you need to cut some paper, use the butcher knife or chainsaw!

This research emphasizes the importance of correct positioning, appropriate teaching of late preterm infants' vulnerabilities, and added vigilance when mothers are primiparous or when the mother's ability to properly assess the baby may be impaired. Late preterm infants are at greater risk for airway collapse because of their decreased tone and immature neurological functioning, so correct positioning and latch are of utmost importance.

SUMMARY

If mothers of late preterm infants were better educated about the benefits of breastfeeding and better equipped with the skills needed to breastfeed these babies, perhaps the cost of medical care and the toll that the medical care takes on families would be greatly reduced. By educating health care professionals about how to overcome the obstacles of breastfeeding late preterm infants, we can equip everyone with the necessary tools to provide age-appropriate care to this increasingly emerging population. Together we can work with the health care industry to provide the best care for these babies, decreasing the mortality, morbidity, and developmental delays consistent with late preterm infants. Not only will the babies be healthier, but so will the mothers of these babies, our health care system, and our environment.

PART II

Conquering Breastfeeding Challenges for the Late Preterm Infant

Prologue

To overcome the myriad complications that late preterm infants can possibly experience, early achievement of effective breastfeeding is of utmost importance. Breastfeeding supplies energy for glucose control, thermoregulation, growth, and normal brain functioning, as well as immunoglobulins for infection control. Colostrum and breast milk can supply all the necessary nutrients almost any baby needs to survive and thrive, but only if it is available and only if we are able to effectively feed it to the infant.

Late preterm infants have historically demonstrated a difficult course of adaptation to extra-uterine life both because of the immaturity of their physiological processes and, often, health care professionals' inability to recognize the extent that these underdeveloped processes have on one another. This lack of normal fetal-to-newborn adaptation interferes with effective breastfeeding, and ineffective breastfeeding has a direct negative consequence on normal adaptation. It is important to take a well-informed approach to caring for late preterm infants to preserve their health and well-being and to maximize their breastfeeding success.

A proactive approach to breastfeeding the late preterm infant is absolutely essential and must be initiated immediately after delivery. A delay in achieving effective breastfeeding and colostrum transfer exponentially increases the risk for both physiological complications and breastfeeding failure. If the late preterm infant is unable to efficiently transfer colostrum at least every 2 to 3 hours, appropriate steps must be taken to ensure sufficient feedings.

Using the techniques and tools for effective breastfeeding, discussed in the second part of this book, nurses and lactation consultants can ensure that the appropriate assistance is given to the at-risk late preterm infant. Assuming the baby will breastfeed when he or she is ready and delaying needed nutrition is a tragic error in judgment.

With even just one unsuccessful breastfeeding attempt, complications are initiated and the normal wiring of the baby is changed, possibly affecting lifelong outcomes.

Late preterm infants are different than full-term infants and the medical community, as well as parents, need to know this. Specific tools and different breastfeeding techniques may be needed to ensure effective breastfeeding with this population of babies until they are closer to term. Although there is definitely a hesitation for lactation professionals to institute breastfeeding tools without adequate visible and measurable indications for use, the late preterm population poses a more challenging scenario. Breastfeeding tools, such as nipple shields, pumps, and supplemental nursing systems, will become commonplace as we evolve to better care for these babies. Instead of viewing these tools as hindrances, we need to change our focus to viewing these tools as any other useful tools we may require in life— something we use to achieve our goal if we are unable to achieve that goal on our own. Tools are temporary, and these breastfeeding tools should be temporary as well, assisting the transition from ineffective breastfeeding of the late preterm infant to highly successful and complication-free breastfeeding of the well-adapted baby, which should be achieved close to the baby's intended due date.

A vigorous baby will wake on his or her own within 1 to 3 hours of the previous breastfeeding and exhibit normal tone, immediate rooting reflexes, sustained latch, strong suckling, and normal initial weight loss patterns followed by predictable weight gain patterns. If the baby is vigorous, no tools are likely to be needed unless there is another underlying complication such as inverted nipples or tight frenulum.

A less than vigorous baby, as often exhibited by the late preterm infant, will need some tools to ensure adequate colostrum and breast milk intake. Each baby should be reassessed at each feeding to see if breastfeeding tools are required. Some babies may require all the tools until they are closer to term gestation, whereas others may need some tools occasionally. It is important that we don't tire the baby with unsuccessful attempts at breastfeeding before initiating the use of breastfeeding tools. It will be evident after two or three attempts to latch whether the baby is vigorous at that feeding. Breast pumps or hand expression should always be used until the late preterm infant proves to be successful at breastfeeding and full breast milk supply is established.

Although this book is specific to late preterm infants, *any* infant having difficulty with breastfeeding can be assisted using the techniques to effective breastfeeding found in the second part of this book.

By assisting the late preterm infant with early, frequent, and effective breastfeeding, we are doing our part to ensure a healthy outcome for these vulnerable, at-risk infants. Gone are the days of triple feeds, uncertainty of effective breastfeeding, and maternal frustration. Using this guide, mothers and health care workers will be more in tune with the needs of late preterm infants and will witness the evolution of breastfeeding success in the late preterm population.

ELEVEN

Health Initiatives

HOW THE LATEST TRENDS IN HEALTH CARE AFFECT THE LATE PRETERM INFANT

Health initiatives are evidence-based policies designed to increase the health and well-being of specific populations. They are usually developed by a collaboration of experts in the particular field of study and prove to be successful in obtaining optimal health outcomes. Two important initiatives for the late preterm infant population are the Baby-Friendly Hospital Initiative and the Late Preterm Infant Initiative.

BABY-FRIENDLY DESIGNATION

One of the latest trends in health care is for hospitals to strive for the prestigious "Baby-Friendly" designation. The Baby-Friendly Hospital Initiative, a worldwide program initiated by the World Health Organization (WHO) and the United Nations Children's Fund (UNICEF) in 1991, encourages and recognizes medical facilities that offer optimal care for infant feeding and mother–baby bonding. The program implements "Ten Steps to Successful Breastfeeding" (Baby-Friendly USA, 2011) and the International Code of Marketing of Breast-milk Substitutes (World Health Organization, 1981) and is a comprehensive and detailed venture aimed at providing excellence in evidence-based maternity care, with a goal of providing the best possible breastfeeding outcomes. The Baby-Friendly status is given only to those facilities that have undergone rigorous training, policy development and implementation, and obligatory auditing.

TEN STEPS TO SUCCESSFUL BREASTFEEDING

The Ten Steps to Successful Breastfeeding were designed to encourage exclusive, long-term, successful breastfeeding. The steps for facilities providing nursing and maternity care are as follows (Baby-Friendly USA, 2011):

1. Have a written breastfeeding policy.
2. Train all health care staff in the skills necessary to implement the policy.
3. Inform all mothers about of the benefits and management of breastfeeding.
4. Help mothers initiate breastfeeding within 1 hour of birth.
5. Show mothers how to breastfeed and how to maintain lactation even if they are separated from their infant.
6. Give newborns no food or drink other than breast milk unless medically necessary.
7. Practice rooming-in, allowing mothers and their babies to remain together 24 hours a day if medically stable.
8. Encourage breastfeeding on demand.
9. Give no artificial teats or pacifiers to breastfeeding infants.
10. Foster the establishment of breastfeeding support groups and refer mothers to them on discharge from the hospital or clinic.

INTERNATIONAL CODE OF MARKETING
OF BREAST-MILK SUBSTITUTES

The International Code of Marketing of Breast-Milk Substitutes was developed in Geneva in 1981 by the World Health Organization (WHO), along with 122 member states representatives, after numerous governments, nongovernmental agencies, professional associations, scientists, and infant food manufacturers called for action to be taken on a worldwide scale to address and improve the health of infants and young children. Through this program WHO has developed methods to increase the rate and duration of breastfeeding worldwide. One of the most important outcomes was recognizing that infant formula should not be marketed nor distributed in ways that might interfere with the protection and promotion of breastfeeding. Through work like the International Code of Marketing of Breast-Milk Substitutes, the Ten Steps to Successful Breastfeeding, and the

Baby-Friendly Hospital Initiative, the international health care community strives to ensure the long-term health and well-being of all infants.

LATE PRETERM INFANT INITIATIVES

Another emerging health care trend is for private and state-funded mother/baby groups, certain professional nursing associations, physician groups, and medical facilities that provide care for late preterm infants to develop and follow what are known as *late preterm initiatives.* These are order sets that focus on providing the most advanced, evidence-based care to late preterm infants to obtain the most desirable outcomes for these babies and avoid the documented common morbidities and mortalities. Late preterm initiatives follow a systems approach, including management of cardiorespiratory issues, metabolic concerns, thermoregulation, neurological status, nutrition and breastfeeding, post-discharge education, follow-up care, and prevention of complications and hospital readmissions.

Probably the most well-known late preterm initiative was launched by the Association of Women's Health, Obstetric and Neonatal Nurses (Medoff Cooper et al., 2012), which included a multi-year education and awareness project related to the nursing care of late preterm infants. It offers a framework of evidence-based practice guidelines for nurses caring for these late preterm babies. Physician groups have begun developing their own late preterm initiatives as well (Hubbard, Stellwagen, & Wolf, 2007), which focus on what the physicians need to implement in order to promote and achieve the best outcomes for these late preterm infants. Working together, nurses and physicians should be able to provide optimal care for these late preterm babies.

In collaboration with many other entities, the National Perinatal Association recently released Multidisciplinary Guidelines for the Care of Late Preterm Infants (available at www.nationalperinatal. org/lptguidelines.php). The guidelines address specific practices aimed at minimizing associated health risks and enhancing care to late preterm infants and represent an evidence-based approach to every aspect of medical care for these infants. They identify specific late preterm morbidities, address medical procedures to reduce the risk of the morbidities, and give appropriate parent teaching for each morbidity and procedure. The guidelines are split into four sections, including stabilizing the late preterm infant, screening for potential risks, safety, and support, and are further broken down into in-hospital assessment and care, transition to outpatient care, short-term follow-up, and long-term follow-up.

DISCORD BETWEEN THE TWO INITIATIVES

One of the most difficult aspects of achieving the best breastfeeding outcomes for late preterm infants is that often there is a clash between the interpretation of Baby-Friendly initiatives and the reality of the challenges involved in providing necessary nutrition to these babies, as evidenced by late preterm initiatives. Unfortunately, two perceived problems exist with late preterm initiatives. First, late preterm initiatives are not always specific in providing guidelines as to *how* to obtain adequate breastfeeding but instead state only the desired outcomes as measurements of frequency and duration of breastfeeding sessions, often with suggestions for use of breastfeeding tools and supplementation aids but not with clear guidelines for their use. Second, the Ten Steps to Successful Breastfeeding guidelines, adopted by the Baby-Friendly Hospital Initiative, were written when late preterm infants were automatically admitted to the neonatal intensive care unit (NICU) or special care nursery until they proved they could feed well on their own, and babies in the NICU were exempt from the strict policies of Baby-Friendly. Now that the late preterm population has shifted from more rigorous, intensive care and monitoring to less supervised and often laidback care from parents and well-intentioned postpartum nurses and pediatricians, guidelines such as "breastfeed on demand" and "give no food or drink other than breast milk" take on a whole new meaning, not necessarily the one intended by Baby-Friendly.

An example of a problem with late preterm initiative guidelines would be if the guideline states, "Breastfeed every 2 to 3 hours on demand." We know from experience that late preterm infants often won't demand feedings at all, but will sleep almost continuously without interventions to wake them and attempt to breastfeed. The initiative, therefore, needs to be specific and detailed, such as, "If the late preterm infant is not waking to breastfeed at least every 2 to 3 hours and is not feeding vigorously at each feeding beginning immediately after birth, initiate the use of breastfeeding assistance techniques such as breast compressions and hand expression of colostrum, and utilize tools such as nipple shields and supplemental nursing systems (SNS) to immediately remedy the poor feeding efforts."

These techniques of breast compressions and hand expression and tools such as nipple shields and SNS will be discussed in the next chapters of this book. They are often an essential part of successfully breastfeeding the late preterm infant.

Step six of the Ten Steps to Successful Breastfeeding, "Give newborns no food or drink other than breast milk unless medically necessary," goes further to provide eligibility guidelines for which particular newborns are deemed excluded from this criteria by virtue of a medical need. These infants to be excluded from this step include babies discharged directly from the NICU, those diagnosed with galactosemia during the hospital stay, those who received parenteral nutrition, and those who were enrolled in clinical trials. Just being a late preterm infant does not qualify an infant for the category of medically necessary supplementation, nor does poor feeding without appropriate interventions.

Appendix B of the Baby-Friendly guidelines has additional infant conditions that may qualify for supplementation of breast milk alternatives. Appendix B presents guidelines based on the definition in The Joint Commission's Perinatal Care Core Measure Set #PC-05 (Milton, 2010). It stipulates three infant conditions and acceptable medical reasons for use of breast milk substitutes. The first two conditions include babies born weighing less than 1,500 grams and very preterm infants born at less than 32 weeks gestation. The third infant condition supports the possibility of necessary supplementation for late preterm infants. It includes "newborn infants who are at risk of hypoglycaemia by virtue of impaired metabolic adaptation or increased metabolic demand . . . such as those who are preterm, small for gestational age or who have experienced significant hypoxic/ischaemic stress, those who are ill, and those whose mothers are diabetic . . . if their blood sugar fails to respond to optimal breastfeeding or breast-milk feeding."

This brings up two compounding issues. First, late preterm infants often do not display *optimal* breastfeeding, even when optimal measures are taken to ensure their success. Second, because of impaired metabolic adaptation and increased metabolic demand, late preterm babies are at risk for several serious health complications, not just hypoglycemia.

Does that mean unless the late preterm baby has a low blood sugar that does not respond to optimal breastfeeding tactics, the Baby-Friendly guidelines do not allow for supplementation with anything other than the mother's breast milk? What about other risks caused by their impaired metabolic adaptation and increased metabolic demand, such as increased weight loss, dehydration, decreased urine and stool output, and increased risk for hyperbilirubinemia? What about the risk that mothers of late preterm infants may not have optimal breast milk supply as a result of lack of effective suckling at the breast?

We must now carefully consider the medical indications for, as well as potential side effects of, supplementation of this population and base our practice on the goals and tenets of the Baby-Friendly Hospital Initiative in order to achieve optimal health for the late preterm infant. Having a documented reason for not exclusively feeding breast milk is our best defense, and striving for optimal breastfeeding tactics immediately after birth is our best strategy.

BEST STRATEGIES FOR OPTIMAL BREASTFEEDING OF THE LATE PRETERM INFANT

Breastfeeding support must be given to each and every late preterm infant, from basic positioning and latch teaching for the possibly vigorous 36-week-gestation baby to the complete gamut of assistance for the typically lethargic 34-week-gestation infant, as well as assistance for the mother in obtaining a full maternal milk supply. Assistance must be given from the first breastfeeding after birth, throughout the hospital stay, and after discharge until that late preterm infant is successfully exclusively breastfeeding without complications.

We must not become complacent and believe that a late preterm infant adequately transfers breast milk just because we witnessed what appeared to be a good breastfeeding attempt, nor should we assume the baby is sleepy and will soon wake up when he or she is hungry. Although some may refer to a sleepy, weakly suckling baby as "lazy," he or she is conserving energy for appropriate adaptation to extra-uterine life. Asking a late preterm baby to take all of his or her feedings without assistance is like having an adult run a marathon without any food or training beforehand. Late preterm infants often exhibit breastfeeding complications later than other preterm infants, so assuming they are effectively breastfeeding without adequate proof is detrimental to both mother and baby's overall health and long-term breastfeeding outcomes.

Be proactive. Start breastfeeding assistance early. Ensure that the mother understands the reasoning behind the need for breastfeeding assistance. Use breastfeeding tools as soon as the need arises. Using a nipple shield at the first noneffective feeding helps maintain the infant's strength and willingness to suckle at the breast. When a mother witnesses effective suckling with a nipple shield, instruct her that at any other breastfeeding attempts without the shield, if the baby is not as vigorous and actively suckling as he or she is at that time, allow for a few minutes of attempts, but then apply the shield to continue the feeding effectively. Appropriate pump vacuum pressures can also be used for a comparison, although pressures can actually be less or more than the actual baby's suckling. Encourage continual breast compressions during feedings until the mother's milk is in and the baby is feeding well without assistance. Skin-to-skin contact is extremely beneficial to both mom and baby, so encourage the mother to continuously "wear" her baby skin to skin until her milk is in and the baby is feeding well. Pumping and hand expression greatly decrease the need for supplementation with breast milk alternatives, so encourage correct and frequent expression of colostrum as well as appropriate techniques for feeding the colostrum to the baby. Offer support to the mother because this will likely be a time of great stress to her and her family, and often simple explanations, along with time frames and goals, help alleviate uncertainty.

The late preterm baby soon will be strong enough to breastfeed effectively all on his or her own, but forcing a baby to do it without assistance when he or she is not yet ready decreases the chances of attaining successful breastfeeding and increases the risk for hospital readmission. Multitudes of late preterm babies have proven their vulnerability, and chances are this one is no different.

SUMMARY

Baby-Friendly Hospital Initiative guidelines and late preterm initiatives greatly increase the health and breastfeeding success of the late preterm infant. Often these initiatives seem to contradict each other in terms of their approaches to achieving their goals. Having clearly defined goals is helpful, but having clearly defined paths to those goals, such as those described in this book, as well as anticipating road blocks, is imperative to obtaining those goals. Combining the two initiatives gives these late preterm infants a fighting chance at becoming successful breast-feeders without the complications often associated with the late preterm infant population.

TWELVE

Early and Frequent Breastfeeding

GOALS OF BREASTFEEDING INTERVENTIONS

Breastfeeding interventions should aim to accomplish three goals: prevent adverse outcomes, establish the mother's milk supply, and ensure adequate milk intake (Walker, 2010). Offering the late preterm infant frequent, effective feedings will help to supply the infant with needed energy for temperature stability and glucose control. Frequent nipple stimulation will help increase the mother's milk supply, and increased milk transfer will help decrease bilirubin levels and decrease weight loss. All these positive outcomes may also prevent unnecessary septic workups in late preterm infants.

FREQUENCY OF FEEDINGS AND EVIDENCE-BASED POSITIVE OUTCOMES

Yamauchi and Yamanouchi (1990) examined the relationship between the frequency of breastfeeding and intake, weight loss, meconium passage, and bilirubin in 140 healthy full-term infants born vaginally without complications. There was a significant correlation between the frequency of breastfeeding during the first and second 24 hours after birth. The frequency of breastfeeding during the first 24 hours correlated significantly with the passage of meconium, minimal weight loss, breast milk intake on days 3 and 5, and acceptable trans-cutaneous bilirubin readings on day 6.

COLOSTRUM: COMPONENTS AND FUNCTIONS

A pregnant woman begins to produce colostrum at approximately 12 to 16 weeks gestation. It is a high-density, almost gel-like substance, which is often yellow because of the beta carotene it contains. The primary function of colostrum is to coat the gut to prevent adhesions of pathogens and to promote gut closure (Verklan & Walden, 2010).

Colostrum contains many substances that protect the body from invading organisms, such as the following:

- Secretory immunoglobulin A (sIgA), which is especially high immediately after delivery and combines with a protein in the mucosa to defend the gut lining from pathogens (*Mosby's Medical and Nursing Dictionary*, 1986)
- White blood cells, especially polymorphonucleocytes
- Lactoferrin, lysozyme epidermal growth factor, and interleukin-10
- Interferon, which has strong antiviral activity, and fibronectin, which causes certain phagocytes to become more aggressive (Walker, 2011)

Colostrum has a mean energy value of 67 kcal/dL (18.76 kcal/oz) compared with mature milk's energy value of 75 kcal/dL (21kcal/oz). Compared with mature milk, colostrum is lower in lactose, fat, and water-soluable vitamins, but higher in vitamins, A and E, carotenoids, protein, sodium, zinc, chloride, and potassium (Walker, 2011).

The laxative effect of colostrum increases the clearance of meconium, thereby reducing bilirubin levels. The goal of early and frequent breastfeeding is to increase the consumption of colostrum, which will decrease the negative effects of poor breastfeeding commonly related to late preterm infants.

ACADEMY OF BREASTFEEDING MEDICINE PROTOCOL #10

The Academy of Breastfeeding Medicine designed a clinical protocol exclusive to breastfeeding late preterm infants. Its goal is to support, promote, and sustain breastfeeding in the late preterm infant and to maintain optimal health for both the infant and the mother.

The purpose of the protocol is multifaceted. It is intended to heighten the awareness of the difficulties that late preterm infants and their mothers have with breastfeeding while allowing the infant to breastfeed and breast milk feed to the greatest extent possible. It offers strategies to anticipate, identify, and manage breastfeeding problems while preventing an array of medical problems associated with poor breastfeeding. It also involves maintaining awareness of the mother's needs, her understanding of the feeding plan, and her ability to cope with the demands of breastfeeding a late preterm infant (Academy of Breastfeeding Medicine, 2011).

The inpatient breastfeeding section of the protocol implements many methods to encourage unlimited, unrestricted breastfeeding, such as encouraging the initiation of breastfeeding within 1 hour of birth and waking the baby to breastfeed if necessary. It further states the infant should be breastfed, or breast milk fed, at least 8 to 12 times per 24-hour period. This inclusion of the words "or breast milk feeding" is very significant. This means that the late preterm infant needs to ingest some colostrum or breast milk at least every 2 to 3 hours. If the baby is unable to latch and transfer colostrum on its own, additional steps by the health care provider or the mother must be taken to ensure adequate feeding volumes. This feeding pattern must begin immediately after birth to decrease the risk of adverse health outcomes, especially adverse neurological outcomes, which can have permanent devastating results.

MATERNAL UNDERSTANDING OF FEEDING REQUIREMENTS: INITIATION OF A FORMAL FEEDING PLAN

Although some people can listen to instructions and follow them well without reminders, the parents of late preterm infants are often overwhelmed by the amount of information they receive immediately after the birth of their baby. Some of this sense of overwhelm comes from lack of sleep as a result of being in labor, overstimulation if the mother has been on bed rest until now, uncertainty about the health status of their infant, and the perception of conflicting messages received from the person delivering the baby ("You have a perfect baby who is breathing on his or her own") and the person explaining the need to hand express and feed the infant ("Your baby is at risk for . . . "). Ideally, the parents would know ahead of time that they are giving birth to a late preterm infant and that this infant will require some specific feeding assistance if not feeding vigorously on his or her own every 2 to 3 hours.

Clear, concise, written feeding instructions should be given to all parents of late preterm infants. This feeding plan should be discussed with the parents after the first or second feeding, ensuring that no more than 3 hours have passed since the beginning of the first feeding and the beginning of the second feeding. Any and all questions about the feeding plan should be answered, and the appropriate method for informing the health care provider or nurse of any problems should be addressed. Encourage the parents to freely seek help if the infant is not feeding effectively.

ANTICIPATE THE NEED FOR ASSISTANCE

The methods for increasing the success of breastfeeding, as discussed in this book, should be employed immediately any time the late preterm infant fails to effectively breastfeed on his or her own. Late preterm infants should breastfeed or receive breast milk at least every 3 hours beginning at birth. Qualitative signs of colostrum transfer are necessary if one is assuming the infant is breastfeeding well. There should be colostrum visible in the nipple shield or on the breast after a feeding, increased swallowing with breast compressions, and very easy expression of colostrum after a feeding. Have the mother attempt hand expression (without the warm compress and massage), performing just one squeeze of the breast immediately after a feeding. If colostrum is not readily available at the nipple tip with one squeeze using proper hand expression technique (see Chapter 18, "Breast Massage and Hand Expression"), it is likely that the infant received very little colostrum during that breastfeeding attempt, and actions should be immediately taken to ensure that a colostrum feeding is ingested.

Anticipation of breastfeeding assistance should be the norm with any late preterm infant, with the goal of assisting the infant until he or she is physically able to breastfeed successfully on his or her own and the mother's milk supply has greatly increased. Inform the parents of the typical late preterm infant scenario with respect to breastfeeding difficulties and the possible need for supplementation, stressing the importance of frequent feedings of colostrum within hours of birth. Give the parents anticipatory guidelines of how to measure effective breastfeeding and when to expect the mother's milk supply to increase, and ensure the parents are aware that any breastfeeding intervention should be temporary until the baby is ready to breastfeed effectively all on his or her own.

SUMMARY

Frequent, effective feedings are the key to health and breastfeeding success for late preterm infants and their mothers. Strategies to improve breastfeeding and breast milk consumption must be employed as soon as the late preterm infant exhibits signs of ineffective breastfeeding. Working together as a team, health care professionals and the parents of the late preterm infants can improve the overall health of the baby, increase breastfeeding success rates, and increase maternal breastfeeding confidence.

THIRTEEN

Decrease Stimuli and Energy Expenditure

THE IMPORTANCE OF DECREASING STIMULI AND ENERGY EXPENDITURE FOR THE LATE PRETERM INFANT

Decreasing stimuli to the late preterm infant is essential for adequate breastfeeding. Overstimulation can negatively affect the baby's respiratory status, his or her awake/sleep cycles, and metabolism and glucose control, and all these negative consequences can have a large influence on the late preterm infant's ability to effectively breastfeed. Decreasing energy expenditure helps to limit excess weight loss, increases available energy for breastfeeding, helps regulate glucose metabolism, and potentially leads to earlier success of exclusive, unaided breastfeeding.

EVIDENCE–BASED RESEARCH: HOW KANGAROO CARE BENEFITS LATE PRETERM INFANTS

Kangaroo care, also known as kangaroo mother care, is defined as constant skin-to-skin contact between a mother and her newborn, allowing frequent and exclusive or nearly exclusive breastfeeding. Introduced in Bogota, Colombia, in 1978 as an alternative approach to traditional neonatal intensive care unit (NICU) care for low-birth-weight infants in response to overcrowded nurseries, scarce and costly resources, and high rates of infection and infant mortality, kangaroo care has since also been shown to improve mother–infant bonding and breastfeeding success (Charpak et al., 2005; Jefferies and Canadian Paediatric Society Fetus and Newborn Committee,

2012). A Cochrane Review, which looked at 16 studies including 2,518 infants, concluded that kangaroo care is associated with reduced risk of mortality, decreased rate of sepsis, decreased risk for hypothermia, decreased length of hospital stay, increased infant growth rates, increased mother–infant attachment, and increased rate and success of breastfeeding (Conde-Agudelo, Belizán, & Diaz-Rossello, 2011).

THE BENEFITS OF MAINTAINING SKIN-TO-SKIN CONTACT

One of the best ways to decrease stimulation and energy consumption is to practice kangaroo care. This constant contact between the mother and her baby decreases external stimuli, reduces baby crying episodes, improves cardiorespiratory status of the baby, decreases energy demand, and improves successful breastfeeding outcomes (Darnall, Ariagno, & Kinney, 2006; Engle, Tomashek, Wallman, & American Academy of Pediatrics Committee on Fetus and Newborn, 2007; Moore, Anderson, Bergman, & Dowswell, 2012; and Raju, Higgins, Stark, & Leveno, 2006). Skin-to-skin contact also stabilizes thermoregulation of the baby, leading to minimal energy expenditure from cold stress (Bystrova et al., 2003), and has the added capacity to increase the mother's milk volume (Hurst, Valentine, Renfro, Burns, & Ferlic, 1997).

Hurst et al. (1997) evaluated the effect of early skin-to-skin holding on 24-hour milk volumes of mothers with ventilated, low-birth-weight infants. Mean milk volumes were calculated at 2, 3, and 4 weeks after delivery. During the 2-week period, the study group showed a strong linear increase in milk volume, in contrast to the control group, which showed no indicative change in breast milk volume. This substantial increase in milk supply is paramount with these late preterm babies, because one of the major difficulties in breastfeeding this population is delayed lactogenesis II (the onset of a copious milk supply, or the milk "coming in").

In a randomized, controlled trial (Hake-Brookes & Anderson, 2008), a sample of 66 mothers and their preterm infants (32–36 completed weeks gestation) who practiced unlimited kangaroo care were shown to breastfeed significantly longer and breastfed more exclusively than the control dyads who did not practice kangaroo care.

Ideally, skin-to-skin contact would begin at birth and continue throughout the hospital stay, at least until the baby is feeding vigorously at each feeding and the amount of mother's milk has increased dramatically. The baby should be placed naked, or just in a diaper, with his or her head covered with a cap, on the mother's bare chest with his or her body embraced in the natural curves of the mother's chest. Although term babies should be placed prone for skin-to-skin contact, placing the late preterm baby prone can lead to respiratory distress, because late preterm infants will not push away from the mother if breathing is impaired. Avoid forcing the head to turn sideways because this can distort the trachea and lead to respiratory distress or arrest. If the baby is unable to turn his or her head sideways on his or her own, place the baby in a more side-lying position against the mother's chest. A warm blanket should then be placed over the back of the baby.

Skin-to-Skin Contact Decreases Negative Stimuli

Not only does constant skin-to-skin contact benefit the baby physiologically, it decreases the amount of negative stimuli to the baby. By maintaining normal body temperatures, the baby does not need to be dressed and swaddled, thereby decreasing the amount of physical movement. The continuous skin contact limits the amount of visitors who come in direct contact with the baby, which might be undesirable to the visitors or the parents but decreases stress to the baby by avoiding excess motion, cold stress, hyperthermia, increased metabolic demand, and light and noise stress, and has the added benefit of reducing the likelihood of acquiring infections from others. The late preterm baby must be made a priority until he or she is physiologically able to positively adapt to extra-uterine life, which may take days to weeks, depending largely on the gestation of the baby.

Skin-to-Skin Contact Increases Mother's Awareness of Infant Feeding Cues

Skin-to-skin contact also helps to increase the mother's awareness of early feeding cues, because late preterm infants often show inconsistency and subtle feeding cues. These cues might involve rapid eye movement under the eyelids, sucking motions of the mouth and tongue, hand-to-mouth movements, wriggling, and slight sounds. If not quickly acted on, these feeding cues may pass and the baby may return to a sleeping state without breastfeeding, or the baby might become distressed and start crying, using valuable energy in the process. As Matthiesen, Ransjö-Arvidson, Nissen, and Uvnäs-Moberg (2001) demonstrated, the movements of the infant's hand act like a massage on the mother's breast, and this combined with suckling and licking of the nipple increase maternal oxytocin release, creating more and stronger milk ejections. Therefore, babies should not wear mittens when skin to skin unless medically indicated.

DECREASE STIMULI TO INCREASE THE LATE PRETERM INFANT'S BREASTFEEDING SUCCESS

Because the self-regulatory system of late preterm infants is often underdeveloped, their response to stimulation may be somewhat unpredictable, with irritability and indifference being demonstrated when parents are most expecting more favorable interactions. Although all babies should experience touch and visual stimulation, especially of their parents' faces, and should hear their parents' voices, the variety and frequency of this stimulation should be limited to one of these activities at a time for a late preterm infant so as not to cause overstimulation. Therefore, when changing a diaper before breastfeeding, for instance, the parent should not talk or put his or her face within arms' length of the baby's face, because this can cause too much stimulation and result in poor breastfeeding.

Signs of Overstimulation in Late Preterm Infants

Signs of overstimulation are often exhibited by either rapid or lower heart rates, abnormal breathing, mottling of the skin, frequent startling, holding the hand in a "stop" position, falling asleep, hiccups, or regurgitation. These cues should be reviewed with the parents so that reasonable expectations of the baby's interactions can be developed (Hubbard, Stellwagen, & Wolf, 2007).

A study published in the _Journal of Obstetric, Gynecologic, and Neonatal Nursing_ (Morrison, Ludington-Hoe, & Anderson, 2006) concluded that there are many interruptions to breastfeeding dyads on postpartum day 1 in hospitals, and these interruptions were perceived to negatively influence breastfeeding, so it would behoove health care professionals to decrease the amount of unnecessary interruptions of these mothers and babies.

Sources of Overstimulation

Constant television viewing, playing loud or continuous music, and multiple telephone conversations should be avoided to decrease noise stimulation to the baby. Lights should be dimmed to decrease visual overstimulation. Rocking chairs may also increase stimuli and stress to the breastfeeding late preterm baby and should be avoided during breastfeeding. The constant motion can be much like being on an amusement ride, causing the baby to become nauseous, or may be too soothing and lull the baby back to sleep during breastfeeding before he or she transfers an adequate amount of breast milk.

As for late preterm babies who are in the NICU, skin-to-skin contact is ideal whenever possible, with constraints as a result of the baby's health status as well as the mother's physical presence dictating this possibility. Luckily, visitors are generally restricted in the NICU and have less opportunity to hold the baby, which benefits the baby by eliminating excess stress and decreasing the spread of germs. Care should be taken to decrease stimuli by keeping monitor alarm levels at a minimum, answering alarms and phones promptly, closing isolette doors carefully, and avoiding placing items on top of isolettes with the baby inside, because the noise from all these can greatly increase stress and negatively affect breastfeeding outcomes.

METHODS TO DECREASE ENERGY EXPENDITURE

Because late preterm babies are born without brown fat stores, they have minimal glucose reserves. This means that even a small amount of excess energy expenditure results in a negative outcome for wake/sleep cycles and weight loss. Several steps can be taken during breastfeeding to ensure adequate energy conservation.

Limit Feeding to One Side If the Baby Is Not Vigorous

Limit feeding to one breast each feeding if the baby is not vigorous and is already being supplemented. Although we were taught to offer the baby both breasts at each feeding, this practice should be limited to term infants or vigorous late preterm babies. For the majority of babies born at 34 or 35 weeks gestation, this practice of trying to latch to two breasts, and the movement and stimulation that comes with positioning them to feed on both sides, is way more than their bodies and minds can handle. The mother's breasts are going to be stimulated by the pump after the feeding, so this does not negatively affect the mother's milk supply, and if the baby is already receiving supplemental feeds, we are assured the baby is receiving enough fluids. If the infant is not receiving supplemental feedings or becomes vigorous during the feeding, both breasts should be offered, ensuring a smooth transition from one breast to the next, limiting stress on the baby.

Limit Duration of Supplemental Feedings

Limit the time of the breastfeeding session when supplementation is being used and the baby is not vigorous at the breast. As noted by the Academy of Breastfeeding Medicine (Protocol #10, 2011), a late preterm baby who is discharged from the hospital should be satisfied after 20 to 30 minutes of breastfeeding. This means the baby should have time to attempt latching and then finish the feeding within 30 minutes. Therefore, with a less-than-vigorous baby, steps should be taken within a few minutes of initiating the feeding to remedy the poor feeding situation, such as using a nipple shield or beginning supplementation at the breast using a supplemental nursing system. Do not allow the baby to become fatigued with latch and suckling attempts before stepping in with the tools needed for breastfeeding success. However, if the baby is vigorous, with or without a nipple shield, or continues to suckle after supplementation is taken, duration of breastfeeding should not be limited, but assistance such as breast compressions should continue to be used to ensure minimal excessive energy expenditure. This is a sign that the baby is becoming more successful at breastfeeding.

Limit Obnoxious Stimuli and Repeated Unsuccessful Attempts

Contrary to the teaching of breastfeeding term infants, long repetitive practice sessions of trying to latch or long times between feedings do not help the late preterm infant perfect his or her breastfeeding skills. Instead, this method has the negative effects of making the breastfeeding experience a noxious one, increases metabolic demand, and increases the risk of hospital readmissions. Although one might think that eventually the baby will wake up and feed when he or she is hungry, evidence has proven otherwise (Adamkin, 2006; Ayton, Hansen, Quinn, & Nelson, 2012; Delaney & Arvedson, 2008; Engle et al., 2007; McDonald et al., 2012; Walker, 2009). The less-than-vigorous late preterm baby initially needs breastfeeding support rather than breastfeeding practice and will have many feedings with which to practice his or her breastfeeding skills when more neurologically mature. Using a nipple shield or a supplemental nursing system will encourage a more effective rate and strength of suckling, providing a much more effective learning session.

SUMMARY

By decreasing unnecessary stimuli to the late preterm infant, the mother is able to provide a nurturing environment, decreasing energy expenditure and creating a more positive experience to the adaptation of extra-uterine life. The energy saved by decreasing excess stimuli can then be used during more awake, alert times, which should lead to better breastfeeding attempts and outcomes. The extremely important skin-to-skin contact will further reduce negative consequences of being born early and will have a positive influence on the mother's milk production. All this should help empower the mother to feel in control of her baby's surroundings and well-being, and lead to a more successful breastfeeding experience for both the mother and the baby.

FOURTEEN

Proper Positioning and Latch Technique

THE IMPORTANCE OF PROPER POSITIONING DURING LATCH WITH LATE PRETERM INFANTS

Improper positioning of a baby at the breast, especially a late preterm baby, can have a huge effect on the quality of breastfeeding. Late preterm infants often exhibit hypotonia, which can lead to poor positioning and ineffective latch. Incorrect positioning can cause inadequate suckling, which leads to delayed lactogenesis II (the significant increase in breast milk production) for the mother and decreased intake for the baby, subsequently leading to hypoglycemia, increased jaundice, and increased risk for dehydration. Improper positioning can also cause increased energy demands, which cause increased weight loss; sore nipples that can lead to decreased frequency and early cessation of breastfeeding; and can even cause apnea or cardiac arrest, especially in hypotonic babies.

CORRECT POSITIONING: THE RESEARCH SUPPORTING THE NECESSITY

When positioning any baby at the breast for breastfeeding, it is imperative that there is adequate extension of the neck to allow for unconstrained breathing. With a late preterm infant, laryngeal reflexes are delayed (Darnall, Ariagno, & Kinney, 2006) and the cartilage is less rigid, causing distortion or collapse of the larynx if there is too much flexion on the head and neck. This may compromise breathing, causing desaturation as well as positional apnea as a result of airway obstruction. Also, the distortion of the trachea leads to distortion of the esophagus, making swallowing difficult, leading to decreased fluid intake and increased risk of aspiration.

Positioning in neutral alignment helps decrease negative responses related to immature autonomic systems. The late preterm infant should be completely supported by a somewhat firm surface, such as a pillow, which will allow adequate length for his or her head to be supported, along with the torso and legs and feet. Alternately, the baby can be positioned directly on the mother's abdomen, being supported by the natural curves of the mother's body. This positioning on the mother's abdomen often works well when mom is obese and the abdomen is able to fully support the infant.

At no time should the late preterm infant's arms or legs be left to dangle, because this can cause the baby to become greatly stressed and has a negative effect on breastfeeding. Dangling limbs during breastfeeding is equivalent to multitasking, which usually results in less than optimal performance, at the expense of breastfeeding. The baby has experienced the sensation of all of his or her body parts being in contact with either other body parts or the womb while in utero, and this change in orientation can be confusing and stressful to the immature late preterm infant.

The baby's head should not be solely supported by only the mother's hand either, but should have a firm stationery surface on which to rest so as to not cause movement of the head after the latch or excess strain on the mother's wrist and shoulder. A folded receiving blanket or extension of the pillow works well for head support.

PRINCIPLES OF OPTIMAL POSITIONING

Many variations of the basic holds may be possible and perhaps needed depending on the mother's condition after birth, but several principles should be adhered to when positioning a late preterm baby for breast-feeding. All these principles allow for optimal airway opening; increased acceptance of spatial awareness for the baby, leading to decreased stress responses; decreased energy consumption; and increased maternal comfort and muscle relaxation needed for appro-priate milk ejection reflexes:

- Position and latch with the chin at a 90-degree angle from the chest.
- The infant should be side lying, head level with and directly facing the breast.

- The infant's nose should be level with the farthest edge of the nipple, so the nipple is not positioned in front of the infant's mouth.
- The infant's head, body, and limbs should be fully supported.
- The infant's arms, legs, and hips should be flexed and in line with the center of the body.
- Baby should be in skin-to-skin contact with the mother.
- Asymmetrical latch ensures that the infant's chin is touching the breast.

This positioning is likely foreign to the mother and perhaps to the nurse as well, because images of breastfeeding babies do not look like this and, especially in the United States, where most people are not accustomed to seeing other people breastfeed, mothers tend to imitate what they perceive to be appropriate infant-holding practices. Unfortunately, most of the images of breastfeeding babies that Americans see are images of older infants and not those of newborns, and very rarely does anyone other than lactation consultants see images of late preterm infants properly positioned and well-latched.

METHODS OF POSITIONING

Football Hold

One of the most effective ways to obtain optimal positioning, keeping all the previously stated principles in mind, is by using a football hold. Ensure the baby is latching using a side approach, not coming up from underneath the breast or from in front of the breast, because both these techniques require flexion of the head and neck, and the weight of the mother's breast on the baby, if coming up from under the breast, can cause severe issues with breathing. A baby lying on his or her back while breastfeeding will have to deal with the added stress of being in a startle position, as well as being forced to swallow in a very unnatural position, which can lead to choking and breastfeeding aversion.

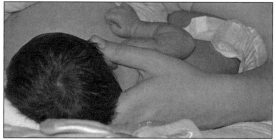

Photo 14.1: A well-positioned baby with flexed extremeties.

The mother should be sitting or reclining comfortably with enough pillows stacked behind her to support her neck, shoulders, and back and to allow her body to be brought out a few inches from the bed. The pillows should be placed vertically behind her so as not to stick out from beside her. This pillow positioning allows the baby's feet to extend out behind the mother while allowing baby enough room at mother's side to be positioned "nose to nipple." Have the mother maintain a forward-facing position with her body and breast, because turning toward her baby will not allow sufficient leg room for the baby, will cause an inappropriate latch with head flexion, and will be uncomfortable for the mother. Remember, the baby is latching from the mother's side.

Place enough pillows beside the mother to allow the center of the baby's face to be level with the nipple. This often entails using a bed pillow folded in half with another pillow opened on top of that. Place the baby on the pillows, on his or her side, with the nose level with the nipple. If the mother has a very long or very wide nipple, the nose should be level with the edge of the nipple that is farthest from the baby's mouth.

Tuck the baby between mom's body and arm, with baby's arms, legs, and hips flexed, allowing as much skin-to-skin contact as possible (see Photo 14.1). Hip flexion is important for trunk alignment, which influences the stability of the head (Redstone & West, 2004). When properly flexed, the baby should have both hands up near his or her neck, with one hand on either side of his or her body (see Photo 14.2). Do not trap one arm down near the abdomen because this can misalign the baby for proper latch. The baby's hands should not be gloved unless medically indicated, because the touch of the baby's bare hands on the mother's breast helps significantly with the

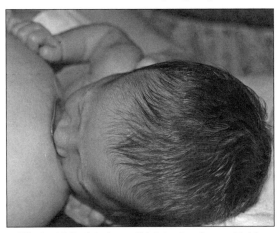

Photo 14.2: A baby well-latched, using a shield. Note the position of the baby's arms on either side of the breast.

milk ejection reflex (Matthiesen, Ransjö-Arvidson, Nissen, & Uvnäs-Moberg, 2001).

Cradle Hold

Mothers often feel the cradle hold, with the baby's head in the crook of their elbow, is the most natural way to hold their baby while breastfeeding. Although it may seem natural to them, it situates the baby in the most unnatural position, causing flexion of the head and neck. The cradle hold may work well once the baby is older and mature enough to know how to reposition his or her own head to find the optimal neck extension, but for a late preterm baby, this position poses several issues. It is difficult to fully support the whole baby with-

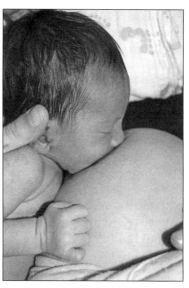

Photo 14.3: A well-positioned, well-latched baby in the football hold. Note the adequate triangle of space between the chin and the chest.

out arms or legs dangling, difficult to allow proper flexion of the limbs and hips, and often the baby is lying flat on his or her back with the head turned toward the breast, causing torsion of the larynx and esophagus, leading to suboptimal breastfeeding and negative breathing outcomes. Adults cannot drink effectively in this position, so why would we expect a baby to be able to do so? A modified cradle hold might be effective if the mother can first position the infant well using a cross-cradle hold and then change the supporting arm, allowing the baby's head to rest on the mother's forearm and not in the crook of her elbow.

Cross-Cradle Hold

The cross-cradle hold might be effective for late preterm babies if the principles of positioning and latch are followed. The baby's body must be fully supported by a semi-firm surface, whether this is with pillows or the mother's body. Positioning nose to nipple is important, and the baby's chin should be 90 degrees from the chest once latched (see Photo 14.3). The baby should *not* be prone with his or her face flat against the mother's breast; this can easily lead to airway occlusion because late preterm babies have decreased muscle tone and immature neurological reflexes and may not lift their head if unable to breathe well enough. Cross-cradle positioning works best when the baby's legs can be positioned and supported lower than the baby's head, usually supported beneath the opposite breast from that being used to breastfeed. The necessary hip flexion of the late preterm infant does not allow for holding horizontally across both breasts because this positioning does not enable the correct chin placement for a correct latch and so may be difficult to achieve in the first few days, especially if the mother is sitting in bed to breastfeed. Once latched correctly using the cross-cradle technique, the mother might find it comfortable to change the supporting arm, essentially ending up in a modified cradle hold with the baby's head supported on her forearm and not in the crook of her elbow. Care must be taken to ensure that the baby's head remains in alignment with his or her body.

Side-Lying Positioning

The side-lying position may or may not work well for feeding a late preterm infant, depending on several factors. It is beneficial in that the baby can be positioned on the surface of the bed or on pillows to be at an appropriate level of the breast; it may be easy to visualize correct infant positioning; and it often allows to mother to be comfortably situated. The drawbacks to this position include the following:

- It is often difficult for larger women to see the baby latch and to visualize correct positioning, which can lead to poor latch or latching to a part of the breast other than over the nipple.
- The mother's nipples might not point in the right direction for optimal latch in this position.
- It may be difficult to achieve optimal skin-to-skin contact, depending on the curvature of the mother's body position, which can lead to hypothermia in a small infant.
- If not done correctly, it immobilizes one of mom's arms and hands, limiting her ability to perform breast compressions or supplementation if necessary.
- It might inadvertently cause the mother to be less cognizant of the baby's breastfeeding progress because she might be more likely to passively breastfeed in this position, and late preterm infants require a more active approach to breastfeeding from the mother.

THE LATCH

Unless part of the baby's face is actually touching the mother's breast, he or she may not know the breast is there or that she is asking him or her to breastfeed. Often babies will grab at the breast with their hands, try to get their hands into their mouths while grabbing the nipple, or push back from the breast. These are all acts of frustration in trying to find the nipple in order to breastfeed. Areolas act as targets so the baby can find the nipple, but the baby can only find the target if the baby is arm's length from the breast, which is not a practical way to start a feeding. The best latch is usually obtained by adhering to the following procedure:

- Without moving the baby from the nose-to-nipple positioning, allow a slight lag of the infant's head, which will position his or her chin on the mother's breast slightly under the nipple. If positioned correctly, this will ensure correct placement of the lower lip and tongue under the nipple, with the correct amount of lip flanging, or "fish lips," without requiring pulling down on the baby's chin once latched. Holding your hand on the baby's shoulder blades, gently guide the baby's head over the nipple once he or she opens his or her mouth. If needing to pull down on the chin more than once to alleviate pinching of the nipple, the baby is likely positioned incorrectly (or may have a tight frenulum), so unlatch the baby and reposition, ensuring a nose-to-nipple placement, with the chin at a 90-degree angle from the chest (see Photo 14.3).
- The stimulus of the chin to the mother's breast should be enough to result in a *full-term* baby opening his or her mouth on cue, but because of the late preterm infant's immature neurological system, this automatic opening of the mouth might not happen right away. Gently moving the baby's face an inch or so away from the breast and then bringing him back to the breast to reattempt the latch might help cue the baby to latch, or gently pulling down on the chin with one finger and waiting for the tongue to drop down to the base of the mouth before gently guiding the baby to latch might be necessary. If pulling down on the chin is necessary for more than a couple of attempts, other techniques such as using a nipple shield might be required until the baby is able to respond appropriately to the chin-to-breast cue. If the baby does not open his or her mouth on cue to the chin-to-breast technique, ineffective suckling may ensue, because the stimulus to latch and suck often go hand in hand. A nipple shield may be needed at this point.

■ Refrain from using either the "sandwich" technique, which squishes the breast using a C-hold, or mouth-to-nipple positioning (as opposed to nose-to-nipple positioning), because both of these usually lead to a symmetrical latch, which results in improper positioning of the nipple in the baby's mouth, which can further lead to ineffective milk removal, nipple pain, and excess energy expenditure.

As noted by Watson Genna and Barak (2010), and Wilson-Clay and Hoover (2005), the chin and jaw placement is the key to correct latch!

Although there is no scientific evidence regarding the need for the mother to hold her breast during latching and breastfeeding, many nurses, lactation consultants, and breastfeeding instructors teach the mother to hold her breast. Aside from having large, pendulous breasts with nipples pointing downward, the reasons for not holding the breast far outweigh the reasons to hold the breast.

First, when mothers hold their breast they tend to move the breast to the baby instead of moving the baby to the breast. This often results in poor positioning of the infant and inappropriate orientation of the nipple inside the infant's mouth. It can also put an inappropriate amount of pressure on the breast in the area of the mother's fingers, which blocks the flow of breast milk, leading to increased risk for blocked ducts, decreased milk transfer, and decreased maternal milk supply.

Second, when the baby is correctly aligned nose to nipple, the baby has free access to the whole breast, but when the mother restricts this access by holding her breast close to the nipple and areola, the baby has to limit his or her latch to the space between mom's fingers and will not push against the fingers to open the mouth wider. This results in a shallow latch, leading to poor milk transfer and, possibly, sore nipples.

Third, holding the breast sometimes makes it difficult to avoid touching the baby's face or lips during the latch. Babies develop the rooting reflex by 32 to 34 weeks gestation, and touching the cheeks, lips, or chin may cause the baby to turn toward the fingers instead of latching correctly or might cause confusion as to where the nipple really is, in which case the late preterm baby can become overstimulated and not be effective at breastfeeding. Because of this rooting reflex and possible overstimulation, stimulation to the baby to elicit suckling once correctly latched should not involve touching the cheek.

While attempting the latch, the mother should have her hands supporting the baby's neck and shoulders and not holding just the baby's head. Be careful that the mother's fingers do not come forward past the baby's ears, as her fingers can elicit the rooting reflex on the cheek and disrupt the latch. Once the baby is properly latched and suckling, the mother can then remove her hand from the baby's shoulder and rest her arm along the baby's back for support (see Photo 14.1). If needed, a receiving blanket can be used for more head support to maintain neutral alignment. Continuous hand support under the head is discouraged because it may cause pain and numbness to the mother's wrist and hand and can increase muscle tension in her shoulder, leading to ineffective milk ejections, decreased milk transfer, and overall dissatisfaction with the breastfeeding experience.

If the baby's nose is compressed against the mother's breast once he or she is latched, *do not* have the mother indent and hold her breast near the nose because this can easily lead to loss of latch as well as blockage of milk flow. Instead, have her use her elbow to bring the baby's bottom and legs in closer to her side or slightly around her back. This movement has a kind of see-saw effect: The legs come in closer, the nose goes out further. This should easily remedy the situation and allow unrestricted airflow to the baby.

TAKE PRECAUTIONS AS NEEDED

Always ensure correct positioning before attempting to latch the baby. A very slight modification to the nose-to-nipple technique might be needed when using a nipple shield. If the nipple shield proves to protrude farther than the baby can easily latch onto with the previously described positioning technique, move the baby slightly forward with a "philtrum-to-nipple" positioning, ensuring, however, that the chin touches the breast when latched (see Photo 14.3).

"Dancer hand" position, using mom's thumb and middle or index finger to support the baby's jaw during feeding, is often a successful technique when bottle feeding late preterm infants. It stabilizes the hypotonic jaw and decreases dead space within the mouth, thereby limiting excess energy consumption. While breastfeeding, however, this technique is not recommended because it can greatly impact the rooting reflex and overstimulate the late preterm infant, leading to decreased suckling responses and ineffective breastfeeding.

The clutch position—often used in the neonatal intensive care unit (NICU) when babies might need to be swaddled during feeds as a result of temperature instability, monitoring equipment constraints, or lack of appropriate breastfeeding-friendly chairs or pillows—should be limited to the NICU setting. The clutch position often does not incorporate correct positioning techniques needed for appropriate breastfeeding responses from late preterm infants and can lead to breastfeeding failure if used outside the NICU on babies who are trying to exclusively breastfeed.

Avoid unpleasant experiences or noxious stimuli while latching, which can include multiple latch attempts, which will impact both the baby and the mother negatively and may lead to breast refusal from the baby or cessation of breastfeeding from the mom.

Refrain from using feeding slings at least until the baby is full term and no longer exhibits signs of hypotonia, because slings can put a disproportionate amount of flexion on the baby's neck and head and can easily result in apnea and death.

Feeding pillows can be used if positioned properly, either around the side of the mother for football hold or across the front of the mother but angled downward for the baby's legs to be below the unused breast when positioned in cross-cradle hold. This placement of the breast feeding pillow is difficult to do while in bed and may be uncomfortable, so it is best used once the mother is out of bed and more mobile. Also, feeding pillows that are designed with a rounded edge as opposed to a flat surface are often difficult to position a small baby on because there is a gap between the mother and the pillow. Rolling up a towel or receiving blanket and placing it in this gap may be useful.

SUMMARY

As noted, correct positioning of the late preterm infant is essential for appropriate breastfeeding. Because of the late preterm baby's hypotonia, slight deviations from neutral alignment can have a drastic negative outcome for breastfeeding success and even the health and well-being of the baby. It is often difficult to teach new latch techniques, but the fundamentals of a proper latch should always be the basis for your teaching. We, as breastfeeding educators, should take a closer look at what we are teaching our patients and how it affects the success of breastfeeding any baby. By correctly positioning and latching the late preterm infant, we are allowing the baby an optimal probability that successful breastfeeding will ensue. By providing the mother with the basics of appropriate positioning and latch, we are enabling her to have the best possible chance at succeeding in breastfeeding her late preterm infant.

FIFTEEN

Breast Compressions

THE IMPORTANCE OF BREAST COMPRESSIONS FOR LATE PRETERM INFANTS

Because of their immature neurological development, late preterm infants often experience decreased frequency and length of wake cycles. Hyperbilirubinemia and resultant phototherapy can further exacerbate sleepiness. In addition, because of the lack of glucose stores and their increased metabolic demand, these babies tend to tire easily and have a great potential for using an excessive amount of calories while breast-feeding. Late preterm infants often have a weaker suck than their full-term counterparts, proving to be ineffective at transferring increasing amounts of colostrum or breast milk. To counteract these challenges during breastfeeding, it is vital that we do all we can to eliminate extra work for the breastfed late preterm baby. As discussed in other chapters, this entails decreasing stimuli, using correct positioning techniques, and using nipple shields, and, as discussed in detail in this chapter, by performing breast compressions. Breast compressions decrease the amount of vacuum pressure necessary to withdraw colostrum or breast milk from the breast, thereby decreasing energy consumption of the late preterm infant.

EVIDENCE-BASED RESEARCH: HOW VACUUM PLAYS AN IMPORTANT PART IN BREASTFEEDING

In a study of intraoral vacuum pressure published in *Early Human Development* (Geddes et al., 2012), results confirm that it is critical for the baby to form a vacuum to remove milk from the breast, and that milk removal does not rely solely on tongue movement along the breast, as once believed. Geddes and her group studied tongue movement and intraoral vacuum pressures of term infants. Using ultrasound images, intraoral vacuum measurements were recorded using both breastfeeding and feeding with an experimental teat that released milk only when a vacuum was applied. The researchers concluded that vacuum is a critical factor in the removal of milk from the breast and that vacuum applied to the breast to remove milk was significantly higher than that applied to the experimental teat (-122 mmHg vs. -67 mmHg). Therefore, we can assume that assisting with the removal of breast milk by use of breast compressions, which can supply colostrum or breast milk to the tip of the nipple, can decrease the necessary vacuum pressures needed for milk removal from the breast, thereby decreasing energy expenditure in the breastfeeding late preterm infant.

Breast compressions are more than just breast massage, although there is likely a similar positive hormonal reaction caused by the mother's hand on her breast (Foda, Kawashima, Nakamura, Kobyashi, & Oku, 2004). Breast compressions are the deliberate compressions of breast tissue done by the breastfeeding mother or assisted by the health care professional, which increase the pressure and flow of colostrum and breast milk within the breast, forcing the fluid out through the nipple at a greater force than if the breast is at rest. More force within the breast means less vacuum pressure needed by the baby to extract the colostrum or breast milk. Because colostrum can be especially thick and viscous, breast compressions can lead to much more effective breast milk transfer, less energy consumption from the baby, and overall increased satisfaction with breastfeeding.

As Pascal's law states, when pressure is exerted on fluid at rest in a closed container, the pressure change is transmitted without loss to every portion of the fluid and to the walls of the container (Pascal's principle, 2013). Although the breast is not quite a closed container, the principle behind the fluid movement is vital to understand here, because improper compressions can lead to a decrease in available breast milk, and the backflow of colostrum or breast milk can lead to blocked ducts or progress to mastitis. Breast compressions can increase the pressure of the breast milk being removed from the breast, requiring less effort on the part of the late preterm infant to transfer the breast milk from the breast.

A study intended to investigate the dynamics of milk removal during pumping (Prime, Kent, Hepworth, Trengrove, & Hartmann, 2012) used a continuous weighing scale to determine changes in milk flow rate over time. Although this study was used to determine something other than what this chapter is discussing, it did demonstrate that multiple milk ejections were detected as increases in milk flow rate, and an increased flow rate was associated with a larger total volume. Using this same principle, the faster the flow of colostrum being removed from the breast, using breast compressions for assistance of flow, the higher the volume of colostrum available for infant consumption.

CORRECT TECHNIQUE INCREASES EFFECTIVE FEEDING AND DECREASES COMPLICATIONS

Many nurses and lactation consultants commonly teach mothers how to do the C-hold of the breast and how to use this hold to compress the breast to stimulate the baby to suckle. Squeezing the breast sends some colostrum or breast milk to the tip of the nipple, enticing the baby to suckle. However, although some breast milk or colostrum is forced from the breast out of the nipple, squeezing the middle of the breast exerts pressure in all directions, including backward into the very ducts we are attempting to drain. This can lead to a continuous backflow of milk, milk stasis, and incomplete emptying of the breast, all of which can have a detrimental effect on milk supply. Also, this form of breast compression, if done close to the areola or baby's mouth, can lead to a change in the angle of the nipple, causing the latch to become less effective or causing the baby to lose the latch completely. Therefore, I don't recommend using this technique often and certainly do not want the mothers of late preterm infants regularly performing this type of breast compression, because compressions will likely be needed for some length of time with these infants and the potential for complications is great.

The most effective way to perform breast compressions is not by squeezing the breast between two or more fingers but by gently squeezing breast tissue between several fingers or knuckles and the ribcage. Compressions are best done by using a fist or three or more fingers, sliding along the breast from the outer edge of the breast tissue next to the ribs, along the breast toward the nipple, forcing breast milk in one direction and out of the nipple. Deep pressure should be applied as the fingers slide over the skin, but not so deep as to cause discomfort to the mother or disrupt the baby's latch. The fingers should stop sliding when they reach about an inch from the nipple. Compressing the breast closer to the nipple than this may cause pressure on the ligaments of the nipple, causing the angle of the nipple to change and the baby to lose a good latch. Once the fingers come within an inch of the nipple, the fingers should be removed from the breast momentarily to allow the breast to refill before sliding the fingers over the breast tissue again from another area of the breast. Compressions should be done along the top and sides of the breast but are difficult to effectively do from underneath the breast without disturbing the baby's latch, so avoid compressions from under the breast. The breast is compressed in the direction from the ribs to the nipple, which helps force the thick colostrum down through the breast to the tip of the nipple. Compressions performed in this manner should not move the breast from its natural position; so if there is excessive movement, instruct the mother not to push so deeply.

These compressions should continue throughout the whole feeding, pausing during suckles if the volume of colostrum or breast milk is too great for the baby to easily manage. It is a good idea to watch the jaw excursion of the baby as he or she suckles; any time the muscles in the jaw stop moving for more than 3 or 4 seconds, initiate a breast compression to remind the infant to keep feeding.

The action of the compressions should increase the rate and strength of the suckling, which should be demonstrated to the mother so that she can observe the effect of the compressions and fully realize the benefit of performing the compressions. Instructing the mother to become aware of her baby's suckling rate and strength during breast compressions is helpful for her to realize how to measure effective breastfeeding. If at any time in the next few weeks the mother assumes the baby is effectively breastfeeding on his or her own, have her mentally compare the rate and strength of suckling unassisted with the rate and strength of suckling during breast compressions. If her baby does not suckle as strongly or as frequently as during breast compressions, breast compressions should be continued.

POSITIVE EFFECTS OF BREAST COMPRESSIONS ON BREASTFEEDING AND MILK SUPPLY

Effective breast compressions are the key to minimizing energy expenditure in the infant while transferring the maximum amount of breast milk during breastfeeding. The more colostrum removed from the breast, the sooner the milk supply will increase. The process of moving the breast milk from the edge of the breast tissue toward the nipple decreases the chance of backflow of milk and maximizes the amount of breast milk available to the baby. I often explain breast compressions to parents this way: Imagine a cup of syrup with a straw in it. Colostrum is thick like syrup, and it takes quite an amount of effort for the baby to suck it up the straw and continue this effort for the whole feeding. Breast compressions help your baby by pushing the syrup to the tip of the straw so all he or she has to do is drink it, conserving energy for your baby. Continued breast compressions allow syrup to be at the tip of the straw at all times and greatly lessens the energy needed to effectively breastfeed.

Although breast compressions require active participation and evaluation on the part of the mother, it is important to realize the positive effect they have on the success of the breastfeeding late preterm infant. Effective breast compressions may increase the baby's fluid intake each feeding, help remind the baby to continue to suckle effectively, decrease the strength of suck needed to remove the colostrum, leading to less energy expenditure and less weight loss or better weight gain, and help to bring mother's milk supply in sooner. By performing breast compressions throughout all feedings until the late preterm baby becomes vigorous at each feeding and no longer needs supplementation, the mother is decreasing the energy her baby needs to breastfeed well, and the baby saves energy stores for growing and gaining weight.

SIXTEEN

Nipple Shields

THE NIPPLE SHIELD DILEMMA: TO USE OR NOT TO USE

Nipple shields are often used in the full-term population for assistance with latch difficulties as a result of flat or inverted nipples or tight frenulums, as a barrier if the mother's nipples are too painful to breast-feed, or to prevent transmission of nipple or areolar infections. In the late preterm population, nipple shields can be used for the same reasons, but more often are used as an aid to decrease the strength of vacuum required from the baby to transfer colostrum or breast milk; to decrease the effects of overactive letdowns, resulting in the infant's inability to control the flow of milk; and as a stimulus to remind the baby to continue to suckle.

Much controversy exists over nipple shield use and their possible harmful side effects. Over the years, nipple shields have evolved from metal, wood, and animal skins, through latex, Mexican-hat style, and bottle teats over the mother's nipples to today's ultrathin silicone version. What is important to note is that the newer silicone shields do not have the same negative effects associated with the others, such as decreased milk transfer, decreased nipple stimulation, and early cessation of breastfeeding.

ULTRATHIN NIPPLE SHIELDS: THE RESEARCH

Although some older studies, such as by Amatayakul et al. (1987) and Woolridge, Baum, and Drewitt (1980), show a decrease in milk transfer while using nipple shields, the newer studies, based on newer ultrathin silicone nipple shields, demonstrate either no statistical difference in milk transfer or an increase in milk transfer when using the shields.

Unfortunately, in a literature review that included articles published between 1980 and 2009, Chevalier McKechnie and Eglash (2010) concluded that all studies they reviewed demonstrated a decrease in milk transfer while the nipple shield was used. However, this is not the case, as the following documented research studies show. Also unfortunate is the lack of current research in the area of nipple shield use.

Researchers Chertok, Schneider, and Blackburn (2006), included in Chevalier McKechnie and Eglash's review, concluded that physiological results demonstrated no significant difference in infant breast milk intake with or without the use of the shield.

Meier et al. (2000) studied 34 preterm infants who used the ultrathin silicone nipple shields to increase milk transfer. They concluded that nipple shield use increases milk intake (18.4 mL vs. 3.9 mL from nipple shield vs. no nipple shield) of breastfeeding preterm infants. All 34 infant subjects consumed more milk with the nipple shield in place than without the nipple shield.

Other research by Bodley and Powers (1996), although not directly measuring milk transfer, confirms that babies who used nipple shields in their study were at or above appropriate weights for those infants at 3 weeks, again at 2 months, and again at 4 months. These babies were not supplemented during the period of nipple shield use.

Clum and Primono (1996) researched how the use of a nipple shield with premature infants affected milk intake and how nipple shield use affects breastfeeding outcome. Complete data was available on 15 of their subjects, between 32 and 39 weeks gestation, who had previously been fed by gavage tube feedings. All these babies had attempted to breastfeed without a nipple shield for an average of 5 days without obtaining a latch or without transfer of breast milk. Although only 9 of the 15 infants (60%) consumed at least 50% of their prescribed feeding amount on their first attempt with using a nipple shield, with two of those consuming at least 100% of their prescribed feeding amounts, those numbers are significant! Zero percent had transferred their prescribed amount of breast milk before the use of a nipple shield, and the transition from gavage feedings to breast feedings is challenging for both the infants and the mothers. Improvement of suckling and milk transfer is usually evident after the first attempt with the nipple shield.

Wilson-Clay (1996) demonstrated that when circumstances occur that may result in disruption or cessation of breastfeeding, nipple shields might be a safe tool to manage effective breastfeeding when other interventions have failed.

Another study (Hanna, Wilson, & Norwood, 2012), using a convenience sample of 81 postpartum mothers in a Baby-Friendly hospital, conducted a structured survey that measured mothers' feelings of helpfulness of the nipple shield, duration of nipple shield use and breastfeeding, and infant weight gain patterns. The majority of the mothers (80%) found the nipple shield to be helpful, with 72% of the mothers indicating it was "very helpful." The median duration of nipple shield use was 6.6 weeks. Breastfeeding duration on average was 12.3 weeks, with 31% of the mothers still breastfeeding at 6 months postpartum, which is higher than the national rate of exclusive breastfeeding of 13.3% at 6 months. It was unknown if these mothers were exclusively breastfeeding or not. The intention to determine infant weight gain using a nipple shield was included in the design of this study, but unfortunately the study did not address this issue directly. Instead, the researchers admit that some mothers gave "low milk supply" as a reason for breastfeeding cessation, but it was unknown if the mothers' perception of low milk supply were accurate or if their perceptions had any effect on infant weights, or if low milk supply was even a result of nipple shield use, because these data were inconsistently tracked by the mothers in this study.

Additionally, an informal telephone survey (Brigham, 1996) of 51 participants who had used a nipple shield for several different latch or suck problems addressed the issues of maternal satisfaction and milk supply. Eighty-six percent of the women reported that the nipple shield helped them to continue to breastfeed and none of them identified insufficient milk supply or poor infant growth patterns associated with nipple shield use.

All these nipple shield studies were addressed by Chevailier McKechnie and Eglash (2010) in their discussion of their literature review as demonstrating "a decrease in milk transfer when the NS [nipple shield] was in place." However, the studies clearly demonstrate otherwise. All the studies had some limitations, and more research is definitely needed to better understand the implications of nipple shield use, but nipple shields should be considered when other attempts at successful breastfeeding have been ineffective, which is often the case with late preterm infants.

Aside from breast milk transfer and infant weight gain concerns during nipple shield use, another concern of nipple shields is whether there is enough nipple stimulation during use to bring in a full supply of breast milk. By measuring prolactin levels and hormonal responses while using nipple shields (Amatayakul et al., 1987; Chertok, Schneider, & Blackburn, 2006) data indicate that hormonal responses with or without nipple shield use are very similar, and therefore nipple shields do not cause a decrease in nipple stimulation as once believed. Studies by Chertok (2009), Chertok et al. (2006), Meier et al. (2000), and Nicholson (1993) all demonstrate that nipple shields do not have a negative effect on the duration of breastfeeding but may actually delay breastfeeding termination.

Although the majority of the studies were not specifically geared toward late preterm infants, the history of nipple shield use and the evolution to a more effective version of nipple shields help reaffirm the value nipple shields can play in breastfeeding babies who otherwise would be ineffective at breastfeeding, including late preterm infants. Although the available research does not specifically describe correct nipple shield application, nor does it state if the nurses, lactation consultants, and mothers actually were instructed on correct application, one must remember that incorrectly applying the nipple shield or incorrect sizing of the shield can have a drastic negative effect on milk transfer, maternal hormone levels, nipple pain and trauma, and breastfeeding experiences.

INDICATIONS FOR USING A NIPPLE SHIELD WITH A LATE PRETERM INFANT

So why is a nipple shield an important tool when it comes to breastfeeding the late preterm infant?

Fat pads in the baby's cheeks help provide an effective seal around the breast and provide stability of the mother's breast in the infant's mouth. Because of the lack of this buccal pad fat, which would have developed after 37 weeks gestation, the late preterm baby has a large area of dead space in his or her mouth. Often the baby will lose contact with the breast and will need frequent re-latching. Until the research presented by Geddes, Kent, Mitoulas, and Hartmann in 2008, it was unclear whether milk was removed from the breast by the peristaltic action of the tongue or via intra-oral vacuum pressure. From their research, it was noted that vacuum plays a significant role in milk transfer from the breast. Geddes et al. (2012) again proved that intra-oral vacuum was the major force behind breast milk removal.

Because of the lack of buccal fat pads, decreased energy stores, and significant sleepiness, late preterm infants often cannot continuously maintain the required intra-oral vacuum pressures over the length of time required to ingest an appropriate amount of breast milk. Minimizing the excess dead space in the mouth decreases the necessary vacuum pressure, leads to decreased energy burning, and increases breast milk consumption. Nipple shields help fill the mouth, decreasing the dead space and thereby assisting the late preterm infant to breastfeed using less energy. Mothers who have very wide or very long nipples might not need a shield because their nipple will fill this space well.

Another appropriate use of nipple shields for the late preterm infant is to control the rate and strength of milk flow from the mother's breast to an appropriate degree for the baby to effectively manage without choking. Some mothers who have a very strong milk ejection reflex, or let down, often find that their babies choke, especially at the beginning of the feedings. Avoiding this situation is crucial to successful breastfeeding. Any adverse reactions causing such an unpleasant experience can create an aversion to breastfeeding and can have a detrimental effect on the success of breastfeeding the baby.

Nipple shields, which have just a few small holes in the nipple tip, allow for the baby to release the milk at a flow that is compatible to the baby's sucking, swallowing, and breathing pattern, thereby decreasing the stress of too fast a flow and allowing the baby to pace himself or herself at the breast. Not only does using a nipple shield in this situation decrease stress on the baby, but it can greatly decrease the stress the mother endures while witnessing the choking episodes her baby experiences with the strong let downs.

The third reason for using a nipple shield when feeding these late preterm infants is to increase the likelihood of the baby having frequent sustained suckling patterns. As research (Larsen & Stensaas, 2003) demonstrates, myelination of the spinal cord does not begin until 36 weeks gestation. Because the late preterm baby's brain has yet to attain the extra layers of myelin, nerve impulses are often lost, so there is little amount of purposeful movement on the part of the baby at this time.

Because the mother's breast tissue is very pliable, it may not give a strong enough impulse to the baby's brain to encourage suckling from the baby. However, the more rigid feeling of the silicone nipple shield and the amount of substance coming into contact with the baby's tongue and roof of his or her mouth encourage much more rapid firing of neurons, which may lead to an increased stimulus to suck.

NIPPLE SHIELD OPTIONS

At the time of this writing, several different options of ultrathin silicone nipple shields are available. I highly recommend using Medela brand nipple shields when breastfeeding late preterm infants. Their design correlates with the principles of nipple shield use for these babies. The size and shape of the nipple part of the shield properly fills the baby's mouth, the shape and length of the nipple part of the shield allows maximum stimulation to the inside of the mouth, the application of the shield to the breast allows for suction to be created and nipple tissue to be drawn into the shield, and the number and size of holes in the tip of the shield allow the baby to properly pace the flow of breast milk or supplementary nutrition. Medela nipple shields come in 16-mm, 20-mm, and 24-mm sizes (see Photo 16.1). Ameda's nipple shield design looks very similar to Medela's design, but it is slightly thicker silicone so should be avoided in the late preterm population. Nuk brand nipple shields have similar-sized holes in the nipple tip and come in a 24-mm size, but their design makes it more difficult for the shield to adhere to the breast.

The designs of other brands of nipple shields are counterproductive to achieving effective breastfeeding the late preterm infant who needs help with breastfeeding, but may be appropriate for use with full-term infants if there is a latch issue because of the anatomy of the mother's nipple. Avent calls their nipple shields "nipple protectors." They have holes in the tip that are too large and allow for a faster rate of flow of breast milk than a late preterm infant may effectively manage. Tommee Tippee

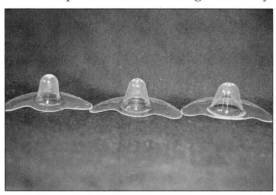

Photo 16.1: Medela contact nipple shields in sizes 16 mm, 20 mm, and 24 mm.

nipple shields also have holes that are too large. Dr. Brown's nipple shields have a short, squared tip that does not allow enough intra-oral stimulation, and it is difficult to achieve a seal with appropriate amounts of breast tissue within the nipple shield.

Regular or Contact Nipple Shields

Whereas most nipple shields just come in a regular design, Medela nipple shields come in two different styles: the regular shield and the contact shield. The regular shield has a completely round rim, and the contact shield has part of the rim cut out to allow the baby's nose to come into contact with the mother's breast, which permits easier breathing because the nipple shield cannot flip up over the baby's nose. It also allows the baby to smell the mother's breast, which usually enhances the rooting and suckling responses of the baby. The regular shield is often easier to use in the first few days of breastfeeding the late preterm infant because it usually maintains better adhesion with the breast and allows for better anchoring of feeding tubes, used for supplementation, inside the nipple shield. However, there are several downfalls of using a regular nipple shield, which must be carefully monitored.

The most common initial reaction of mothers using the regular nipple shield is to become overly anxious about whether or not the baby can breathe, and often the mother will inadvertently remove a large amount of breast tissue and nipple from the baby's mouth to create a large gap around the baby's nose. It would behoove anyone initially demonstrating nipple shield use to a mother to include the following information *before* attempting to latch a baby to the breast using a regular nipple shield:

- If you can see a nostril, the baby can breathe. If the nipple shield rim flips up and over the baby's nose, it does not "saran wrap" to the nose, but still allows air to circulate, and you have time to carefully pull the rim back down.
- If it is necessary to hold the rim of the nipple shield down, hold it down using one finger on the breast at the level of the baby's nose, with just enough pressure to allow contact of the nipple shield with the breast, but not with so much pressure as to indent to breast, because that can cause decreased milk flow and lead to blocked ducts.

- Holding the rim down at the level of the baby's nose allows more airflow around the nostril, but holding the rim down at the level of the baby's mouth removes breast tissue from the baby's mouth and decreases milk transfer.
- Sometimes applying a very light film of lanolin breast cream to the nipple shield rim helps to create adhesion of the shield to the breast, but too much cream will cause the shield to move.

Alternately, a contact shield can be used, and I recommend using this type of shield if nipple shield use is anticipated for more than a couple of days. Follow the same principles as using a regular nipple shield. Using the contact nipple shield can enhance the mother's experience with using a nipple shield. The fear of the nipple shield blocking the baby's airway and the awkwardness of holding the rim of the shield down are eliminated when using a contact nipple shield as opposed to a regular nipple shield.

CORRECT NIPPLE SHIELD APPLICATION

Correct Sizing

The two paramount details about using a nipple shield are to make sure it is applied correctly and that it is the correct size for both the mother and baby. If incorrectly used, there will likely be considerably less milk transfer, increased nipple pain, and, possibly, visible nipple damage. In addition, the baby may expend a large amount of unnecessary energy trying to obtain an adequate amount of breast milk, leading to fatigue and weight loss. If the shield is too big, the baby might have difficulty latching deep enough without gagging and will likely take a shallow approach to the latch, which will affect milk transfer and maternal nipple comfort. If the nipple shield is too small, the mother's nipples might not fit in the tip and there definitely won't be enough breast tissue for the baby to latch onto, which will decrease the amount of milk transfer and increase nipple pain. Also, if the shield is too small, the baby learns to close his or her lips around the tip tightly, instead of learning to open his or her mouth wide, as needed to appropriately breastfeed at a later time without the shield.

The largest nipple shield that suits both the baby and the mother should be used. If using a shield other than the largest 24-mm shield available, attempts should be made every few days to advance to the larger size, and once the baby graduates to using the larger size, he or she should not go back to using the smaller one. Although the old packaging of nipple shields used to have a measurement guide on the back, which one could use to measure the base of the mother's nipple to determine the correct size nipple shield needed, this practice is no longer deemed appropriate and the nipple shield manufacturing companies have discontinued these guides. In addition, at the time of this writing none of the companies who manufacture nipple shields have sizing instructions on the nipple shield packaging, nor do their websites offer instructions on correct sizing. Instead, they defer to issuing a statement that nipple shield selection and use should be in conjunction with professional lactation advice. Therefore, it is of utmost importance to learn how to choose the correct size, know how to correctly apply the nipple shield, and be prepared to fully educate the mother on both of these aspects of nipple shield use.

Applying the Nipple Shield

Application of the nipple shield is easy after practicing a couple of times, following correct application technique. Although the packaging of the nipple shields includes application instructions, the instructions are often confusing, so I have attempted to break down the process in a much more user-friendly way. I have also adapted the process to allow mothers with long fingernails to be able to appropriately apply the shield and still allow an increased amount of breast tissue within the shield, leading to more effective use.

- Ensure the nipple shield is clean before use. It should be washed with hot, soapy water and then rinsed with hot water. Wetting the shield with hot water before use may make it more pliable and easier to adhere to the breast.

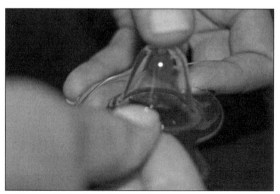

Photo 16.2: Start by pushing down on the nipple part with your thumb, while pulling up from the bottom with your fingers.

■ Turn the nipple shield *halfway* inside-out by placing one thumb flat over the tip of the shield and applying even pressure downward with the thumb as you fold the shield up from the bottom using both hands with fingers on the rim of the shield (see Photo 16.2). The nipple shield should be able to stay in this position without flipping back (see Photo 16.3). Don't poke the tip down with the tip of the thumb because this will turn the nipple shield the wrong way out.

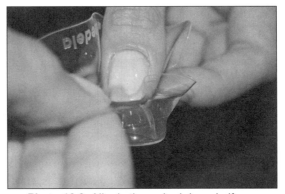

Photo 16.3: Nipple tip pushed down halfway.

■ Place the tip of the nipple shield centered over the tip of the nipple, pushing into the breast gently but firmly to create a seal (see Photo 16.4).

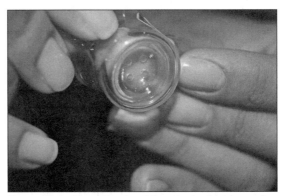

Photo 16.4: Place the tip of the nipple shield over the nipple.

■ While pushing gently into the breast, insert a finger from each hand into the ridge between the nipple part of the shield and the outer part of the shield. Fingers should be parallel to the nipple (see Photo 16.5).

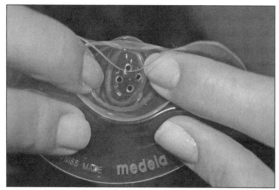

Photo 16.5: One finger from each hard inserted into the ridge.

■ Use your fingers to apply gentle pressure to the bottom of the nipple, going from parallel fingers and nipple to perpendicular fingers to nipple (see Photo 16.6). This should cause the shield to flip itself right side out and draw both nipple and breast tissue into the shield.

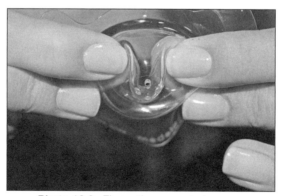

Photo 16.6: Finger tips move to be more perpendicular, causing the tip to flip out.

■ Occasionally the nipple part of the shield won't flip out on its own, so wiggle it gently in a clockwise or counterclockwise direction until it pops out. Do not pull up on the tip of the shield because this might allow air to get in the tip and disrupt the seal.

- Do not just stretch the shield over the nipple because doing so may not create enough suction to draw in enough breast tissue.
- The idea is not to smooth out the rim of the shield but to have the shield fold itself right side out as it makes contact with the nipple and areola, drawing nipple and breast tissue into the tip.
- Ensure that there is at least some breast tissue and not just nipple in the shield. The breast tissue might be wrinkled, but that is okay. Try to get as much breast tissue as possible into the shield.
- If the suction on the nipple and breast is lost at any time, reapply the nipple shield using the previous steps.
- To remove the nipple shield from the breast, peel from the outer rim. Don't pull up on the nipple tip because this can cause pain and damage the nipple.
- Nipple shields are reusable and can be moved from one breast to the other. No need to wash between breasts unless otherwise medically indicated (for example, when the mother has a skin infection on one breast, in which case it would be better to have a separate nipple shield for each breast), but ensure that it is washed before the next use.

To view an online video of the appropriate technique for nipple shield application, go to YouTube (www.youtube.com/watch?v= gIUgmdF6jJM) and watch "How to Put on Nipple Shields."

APPROPRIATE LATCHING

Babies should be allowed to attempt to latch and suckle at the breast before nipple shield use. If unable to maintain a latch and effectively suck, limit the attempts to just a few minutes before initiating the use of the shield. Too many latch attempts with a late preterm infant will cause exhaustion and may cause an aversion to the breast. Ineffective suckling will lead to further fatigue, increased weight loss, and feelings of maternal inadequacy.

To ensure the baby latches properly, the baby should be encouraged to open his or her mouth as wide as possible. This can be achieved using three different techniques:

- Position the baby's nose to the tip of the nipple shield and allow the head to tilt back slightly so the baby's chin touches the breast just below the nipple, encouraging a rooting reflex, which may or may not be present in a baby of this gestation.

- Gently apply downward pressure to the chin with one finger and wait for the baby to drop his or her tongue down and fully open the mouth.
- Hold the nipple shield using a C-hold and gently tickle the baby's lips until he or she opens the mouth; then quickly pull the baby onto the nipple shield. Ensure that using the C-hold does not interfere with the suction created inside the shield or the nipple shield will have to be reapplied to obtain this suction.
- The last two methods of latch should not be used *without* the nipple shield because they result in an ineffective symmetrical latch and can result in the nipple being at the wrong angle in the baby's mouth.

Bring the baby as close as possible to the breast, ensuring that both the chin and upper lip are touching the flat part of the nipple shield, which is touching the breast (see Photo 16.7). The baby should be latched onto the breast tissue that is inside the nipple shield and not just onto the nipple. If there is a gap between the lips and breast, it is likely that the baby will expend more energy than should be required for appropriate breastfeeding. Sometimes a slight position change, moving the baby around the mother's body so the baby's head is slightly extended, allows for a better latch with the chin touching the breast.

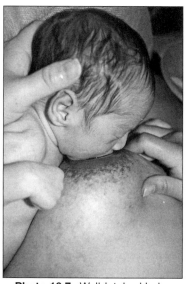

Photo 16.7: Well-latched baby using a nipple shield.

Most late preterm infants will be able to use a 24-mm nipple shield if they weigh at least 4½ pounds. Initially the baby might gag a few times as he or she works out the correct positioning of the tongue. Allow the baby time to adapt to this new sensation. If he or she continues to gag, use a smaller shield if appropriate and return to the larger size after a few feedings.

Use the nipple shield for every feeding, after a short attempt at latching, licking, and suckling without the shield, until the baby is actively rooting at feeding times and has been feeding well with the shield. A baby born at 36 weeks gestation might be vigorous enough at most feedings and not need a shield for the majority of feeds, but it's good to have a shield ready and know how to use it for those few times the baby is tired, doesn't latch well, or doesn't maintain active suckling for at least 15 minutes. A general rule of thumb is that late preterm babies often need the nipple shield until they are about 37 weeks or weigh about 7 pounds, and then they might require occasional use until they are full term, but do not discontinue the shield if the baby is not ready.

WEANING FROM THE NIPPLE SHIELD

There are two ways to wean from using the nipple shield once the baby has become a good breastfeeder and is ready and strong enough to try without it. The first is to try to latch the baby to the breast without using the shield at all. This is a good thing to try if the baby is alert and eager at feeding time. If the baby can't maintain a good latch and suck appropriately for at least 15 minutes, then apply the shield and continue the feeding. You should be able to witness strong, long jaw movements during the feed with only minimal pausing between sucks. Please don't wait until the baby is too tired before reapplying the nipple shield if needed, because practice without the shield is only appropriate if the baby can transfer the necessary amount of breast milk without tiring.

The second way to wean from the nipple shield is to start the baby with the shield on. After a couple of minutes of vigorous suckling, quickly remove the shield and re-latch the baby without it, remembering to correctly position the baby before re-latching. If the baby is unable to latch and suck well for at least 15 minutes without the shield, please reapply the nipple shield. Multiple attempts to wean using this method throughout one feeding can be very confusing to the infant, so if the baby is unable to continue appropriate suckling without the shield after the first removal attempt, reapply the nipple shield and attempt weaning the shield at a later feeding.

IMPORTANT PRECAUTIONS

Just a word of caution when using nipple shields. As a result of the way the nipple shield is constructed, it is difficult for the baby to get a deep enough latch to include much areola, because he or she is limited to the amount of tissue in the tip of the nipple shield. Over time, this can lead to plugged ducts and mastitis. This is one reason for using the largest nipple shield possible; it allows for more breast tissue in the baby's mouth and better breast drainage. Often breast compressions or massage during feedings help prevent plugged ducts from occurring. Also, ensure that the mother is not continually indenting the breast if holding the shield during feedings. There are other causes of blocked ducts as well, but we want to ensure we are not adding to this possibility by inadvertently blocking the natural flow of breast milk from the breast.

Mothers with doorknob-shaped nipples may not be able to use nipple shields because the shape of the nipple may prevent proper suction to the breast during application. If this situation arises, it is likely that the nipple is large enough to fill the late preterm infant's mouth for effective breastfeeding, but diligence to proper latch is essential.

Mothers should be taught the correct way to apply the nipple shield, encouraged to use appropriate methods for cleaning and storing the nipple shield as the manufacturers suggest, and to recognize signs of complications, such as using a shield that is too small or developing blocked ducts. They should also be encouraged to follow hospital protocols for obtaining regular weight checks for their babies to ensure appropriate weight gain while using the nipple shield and given appropriate information about where they can obtain help with breastfeeding once they are discharged from the hospital.

SUMMARY

Although it might seem like a lot of work for the nurse to teach the mother correct use of a nipple shield, and it may initially be frustrating for the mother to have to use a nipple shield and practice correct techniques, nipple shields do play a very important role when it comes to breastfeeding the late preterm infant. Using a nipple shield helps conserve the baby's energy, encourages stronger and more frequent suckling, and controls the rate of milk flow to an acceptable level for the baby. By watching her late preterm baby breastfeed effectively with the nipple shield, a mother may feel more in control of her ability to perform what she believes to be the most natural basic instinct, which encourages continued breastfeeding. With a little time, practice, and patience, the late preterm baby will be ready to be weaned off the shield and will progress effortlessly to successful, uninhibited breastfeeding.

SEVENTEEN

Breast Pumps

WHY CONSIDER A BREAST PUMP FOR THE LATE PRETERM INFANT?

Because of the immature neurological development of late preterm infants, the strength of suckling and stamina for sustained suckling at the breast is often greatly diminished or perhaps even nonexistent. This lack of effective suckling interferes with milk transfer and with nipple stimulation, and consequently negatively affects maternal breast milk production. Even with a vigorous late preterm infant, one should not assume adequate nipple stimulation from breastfeeding alone to bring in a full supply of breast milk, because the visible effort exerted often does not match the results of milk transfer, and late preterm babies can trick even the most experienced lactation consultants into believing they are breastfeeding well.

The first few days, and especially the first 2 weeks, are the most important time to establish milk supply. Delay in breast milk establishment has a long-term effect on overall supply and could result in the necessity of supplementation of the baby, perhaps long term, further inhibiting successful breastfeeding. Therefore, all mothers of late preterm infants should be taught how to pump their breasts and encouraged to be proactive in this form of nipple stimulation until the baby is able to establish and prove effective, successful breastfeeding on his or her own.

UNDERSTANDING BREAST PUMPS: THE BASICS

With so many types of pumps available to consumers, how do you know which pump to recommend to parents of late preterm infants? What if they have already purchased or borrowed one and want to use that one? Often lactation consultants will suggest renting a pump for the first few weeks until the mother's milk supply is well established and then recommend using the pump the mother has already purchased. Why? Rental pumps, intended as multiuser pumps, are different than personal-use pumps in terms of their ability to produce and maintain a full milk supply. It is important to use a pump that has research-based evidence of effectiveness to bring in a full milk supply independent of whether or not the baby is breastfeeding well. Single-user pumps have not been proven to achieve this goal.

FDA REGULATED

Breast pumps, like any other medical device, are regulated by the Food and Drug Administration (FDA) in the United States. Although some pumps are labeled "hospital grade," the FDA does not recognize this term (FDA, 2013) because there is no consistent definition, and consumers need to know that the term *hospital grade* does not mean it is safe or hygienic, as manufacturers would like you to believe. Instead, the FDA encourages manufacturers to use the terms *multiple users* and *single user* in their labeling but does not regulate this. Terms such as *multiuser* and *single user* are definitions that the manufacturer specifies when they register the device with the FDA. Multiuser pumps must have some barrier to ensure there is no cross-contamination from users, and each user must have their own

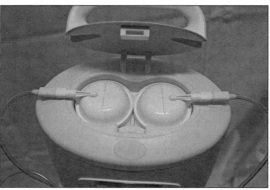

set of accessories (see Photos 17.1 and 17.2).

Medela, a leading manufacturer of breast pumps, defines *hospital grade* as designed for multiple users and having special barriers and filters to prohibit milk from entering the pump motor, which prevents cross-contamination; in

Photo 17.1: Medela pump with multiuser filters.

addition, it guarantees that the motor is as effective as if it were brand new (Medela, 2013). Limerick, Inc. (2013), another leading manufacturer of multiuser hospital-grade pumps, gives the definition of *hospital grade* as effective, evidence-based, and shown to establish a milk supply in pump-dependent women; safe, with features that will

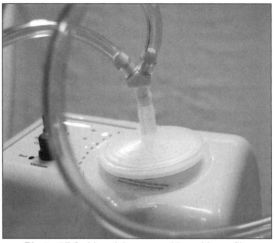

Photo 17.2: Limerick pump with multiuser filter.

minimize the risk for nosocomial infections, cross-contamination, and reinfection; durable; and meeting electrical requirements established by hospitals.

Single-user pumps, like other electronic gadgets, often wear down over time, and the motor is usually only guaranteed for 1 year. A single-user pump cannot be returned to the retailer once used, because infectious diseases have the potential to be spread through sharing these devices.

EVIDENCE-BASED RESEARCH ON BREAST PUMPS AND THE PREMATURE INFANT

Breast pump manufacturers have done some excellent research into the efficacy of their pumps in terms of the ability to establish and maintain a full milk supply in pump-dependent women. The research has been done mainly with mothers of very-low-birth-weight infants in the neonatal intensive care unit (NICU), who are not directly breastfeeding because their babies are too small, too weak, and too ill.

Medela and a research team from Rush University Medical Center, led by Paula Meier (Meier, Engstrom, Janes, Jegier, & Loera, 2013), realized that breast pumps could only simulate the nutritive sucking pattern of a healthy infant during mature lactation, after the milk supply had been established. However, in the first few days after birth, while maternal milk supply is limited, infants suck more irregularly with rapid sucks and longer pauses. This knowledge led to the hypothesis that this type of suckling pattern may be critical in the establishment of adequate milk volume and to the realization that pump-dependent mothers do not have an infant to stimulate their breasts in this very different manner. This encouraged the team of researchers to investigate and evaluate numerous pumping patterns that replicated the suckling patterns of the newborn infant.

They conducted a blinded, randomized clinical trial with 105 breast pump–dependent women of premature infants. One group of mothers used the standard pumping pattern for the whole trial, and another group used a modified pattern, simulating the suckling of a newborn infant before lactogenesis II (the onset of copious milk supply, or milk "coming in"), then switching to the standard pattern once their milk had come in.

The group with the modified pumping pattern, now known as the Preemie 1.0 card, had milk output that was significantly greater than that of the group using just the standard program, Standard 2.0 card. Mothers who used the Preemie card program and switched to the regular card only after the attainment of lactogenesis II reached the same volume of milk production as term mothers by day 6 and matched their milk volumes through the remainder of the 14-day trial period. At day 6, milk volume was between 500 and 600 mL/24 hours of pumping for the Preemie card users and only between 300 and 400 mL/24 hours of pumping for the Standard card users. At day 14, milk volume was between 600 and 700 mL/24 hours and between 350 and 500 mL/24 hours for Preemie and Standard card users, respectively.

Also interesting to note from this study is that, on average, the mothers using the Preemie card before switching to the Standard card had much more efficient output per minute, allowing them to pump 124 fewer minutes during the first 14 days. The implications of this multiphase pumping process on the effectiveness of milk production in the late preterm population are astounding!

Ameda, another manufacturer of breast pumps, tested its Elite pump against milk volumes produced by the Medela Symphony 2.0 card, the Preemie 1.0 plus Standard 2.0 card, and healthy breast-feeding babies (Ameda, 2013). The Elite consistently produced more milk than either of the Medela pumps and by day 5 surpassed the breast milk volumes of the healthy breastfeeding babies. Not only did it produce minimum milk volumes needed, it was demonstrated to achieve full milk production, ideal for long-term exclusive breast-feeding. The Elite, which has multiphase pumping, also has the benefit of being able to make even minor adjustments to the vacuum and frequency of cycling, allowing custom tailoring of the pump settings to best meet each individual mother's comfort and respond to each of her body's needs.

These results were similarly reproduced by Larkin, Kiehn, Murphy, and Uhryniak (2013) using a nonexperimental, descriptive study of 26 mothers who delivered premature infants between 26 and 32 weeks gestation. The mothers used the Ameda Platinum breast pump, a more recent version of the Ameda pump, exclusively eight times daily for 14 days. The average daily milk volume was 817 mL/day for all mothers, with 16 mothers producing more than 700 mL/day and 9 of those mothers expressing more than 1,000 mL/day. Mothers producing the least amount of milk (less than 500 mL/day) used higher suction pressures, faster ending speed cycles, and longer pumping times. This reinforces the need for pumps with separate controls of speed and suction, allowing the mother a wide range of options to achieve greater comfort and more milk ejections, leading to optimal milk expression. The results also reinforce the need for proper education about the importance of maternal nipple comfort during pumping to achieve maximum breast milk output.

PJ's Comfort pump, manufactured by Limerick, Inc., is another pump demonstrated to achieve full milk supply in pump-dependent women (Limerick, 2013). In a nonblinded, prospective trial, a convenience sample was compared with recent historical controls in a similar population of preterm infants in a community level III NICU during a 24-month period. The objective was to determine if mothers would be able to establish an adequate milk supply, comparable to that achieved with more expensive breast pumps, but with a compressible silicone flange. The results showed that 83% of mothers achieved 350 mL/day or more, 66% of mothers achieved 500 mL/day or more, and 29% of mothers achieved 700 mL/day or more. In addition, comments regarding comfort, ease of use, and pump features were all very positive. Milk volumes obtained using PJ's Comfort breast pump were equal to or better than those of other more expensive breast pumps and met or exceeded adequate milk supply in pump-dependent women.

The EnDeare pump (Hygeia, 2013) is another multiuser pump with the same 250 mmHg vacuum as other multiuser pumps and independent speed and suction controls, allowing for multiphase pumping. The ability to customize these controls allows for maximum efficiency and maternal comfort. Although Hygeia does not offer any independent research into their product, the specifications mimic other multiuser pumps that have proven effective in establishing a full breast milk supply in pump-dependent women.

HIGHER STANDARDS FROM PUMPS
FOR LATE PRETERM INFANTS

Because late preterm infants are unpredictable in the rate and strength of suckling and their ability to effectively breastfeed and establish a full milk supply, the mothers of these babies should be instructed on the importance of using a pump that has a proven track record, such as those described previously. When educating parents about the different types of pump required for a mother of a late preterm infant and how each type affects breast milk supply, the standards that need to be adhered to are as follows:

- Multiuser pump with features that eliminate the risk of nosocomial infections, cross-contamination, and reinfection
- Electric, automatic cycling, double pump with varying frequency and pressure controls
- Evidence based, shown to establish or maintain a sufficient milk supply in pump-dependent women

PUMPING STYLE AND EFFECT ON SUPPLY: RESEARCH,
OUTCOMES, AND EVIDENCE

Simultaneous pumping (both breasts at the same time) should be encouraged over sequential pumping (one breast and then the other) because it has been shown to produce a significant increase in milk production (Auerbach, 1990; Hill, Aldag, & Chatterton, 1996; Jones, Dimmock, & Spencer, 2001; Prime, Kent, Hepworth,

Trengove, & Hartmann, 2012) and cuts pumping time in half. Jones et al. (2001) demonstrated the following milk expression amounts on 36 women with preterm infants in a NICU in the United Kingdom:

- Sequential expression without massage: 51 grams
- Sequential expression with massage: 79 grams
- Simultaneous pumping without massage: 88 grams
- Simultaneous pumping with massage: 125 grams

The massage occurred before pumping, but theoretically, additional massage during pumping could even have higher yields.

Several studies comparing pump expression, hand expression, and exclusive breastfeeding have caused some confusion over the best approach to take when dealing with late preterm infants. Keep in mind that most of the studies were done with healthy term babies and their mothers, where the issues of suckling strength, frequency, and the effect on maternal milk supply do not resemble those of the late preterm population.

Interestingly, in one study, breast pumping between 24 and 72 hours after cesarean delivery did not improve milk transfer in the infants studied, and it had a negative effect on the duration of breastfeeding in primiparous women (Chapman, Young, Ferris, & Pérez-Escamilla, 2001). When compared with hand expression in another study, initially the median volume of milk expressed was more for pumping mothers (0–5 mL vs. 0–40 mL), but at 2 months the mothers who were hand expressing were more likely to still be breastfeeding than the mothers who were pumping their breasts (Flaherman et al., 2012). Another study showed that mean basal levels of prolactin in multiparous women were lower than in primiparous women but milk transfer was greater in these multiparous women, implying that milk production is dependent on prolactin receptors in the breast (Zuppa et al. 1988) and not circulating prolactin levels, whereas Jones et al. (2001) concluded that prolactin bioavailability is significantly lower in mothers who deliver prematurely. Chatterton et al. (2000) demonstrated that stress interferes with milk production in mothers of preterm infants. Finally, Leonard, Labiner-Wolfe, Geraghty, and Rasmussen (2011) demonstrated that in overweight or obese women, those who had ever expressed their milk had longer durations of breastfeeding than did those who never expressed milk.

CLINICAL SIGNIFICANCE OF PUMPING RESEARCH

Appropriate Use

So what does all this research really mean, and how does it affect the late preterm infant and the breastfeeding mother? Although routine pumping should not be initiated for all healthy, term infants, it should be included in the feeding plan of all late preterm infants because the reasons for and effects of pumping are different in this population. The mother should be properly educated about why pumping should be initiated and continued; what effect pumping has on her milk supply; how often pumping should be done, and for how long pumping should be performed at each session; effective ways to supplement her baby with the expressed breast milk; breast milk storage guidelines; and appropriate goals that need to be obtained before cessation of pumping. Because breast milk storage guidelines occasionally change, I have not included them here but urge you to refer to the latest guidelines published at www.womenshealth.gov/breastfeeding.

Early and Frequent Expression

Mechanical pumping of the breasts should begin early and be done frequently to increase prolactin (basal or receptor sites), which is necessary for milk production. Simultaneous pumping with breast massage should be encouraged over sequential pumping to increase immediate and long-term milk supply. Mothers should be educated about the fact that over the first 2 to 3 days, *visible* effects of mechanical pumping may not be present but physiological effects are occurring, setting the stage for an adequate or abundant milk supply. It is also very important to acknowledge, especially with primiparous women, that pumping is a *temporary* procedure until her milk supply is established and her baby has proven to be effective at breastfeeding. There should be collaboration between nursing staff or lactation consultant and the pediatrician to develop this plan, keeping in mind that it may need some minor revisions once mother and baby are discharged from the hospital, such as the specific desired weight to attain before cessation of pumping (often a pediatrician-specific measurement) or the rate of weight gain needed before cessation of pumping occurs.

Correct Setup and Use

Mothers of late preterm infants should be properly instructed on the setup, use of, and cleaning of a multiuser, hospital-grade, double electric breast pump that has a proven track record to fully establish milk supply, and should have unlimited access to the pump at least while in the hospital. Staff should assess for correct pump flange (the piece of the pump that actually touches the breast during pumping, also called a breast shield) fit and appropriate vacuum pressure, and ensure that the mother understands the assessment of these two variables, because nipple size and pliability may change over the course of pumping. Hospital staff should be able to assist the mother with the procurement of an effective breast pump before discharge for use at home if her baby is not yet effectively breastfeeding, if the mother's milk supply has not yet greatly increased (lactogenesis II), or if supplementation outside the hospital is needed, all of which are quite likely in this late preterm population.

GUIDELINES FOR CHOOSING A BREAST PUMP AND USING IT CORRECTLY

Proper use of the pump is pivotal in its success or failure, on the comfort of the mother, and ultimately on the adherence to the treatment plan. The pump should be comfortable to use, not causing any pain or discomfort to the mother. Nipple pain during pumping will have a negative effect on supply, either through the autonomic system in which painful pathways are interrupted (the nipple telling the brain "I don't really want to do this"), or through the direct cause of the pain itself interfering with milk expression (rubbing and constriction of the nipple, blocking the flow of breast milk).

There are two main types of double electric breast pumps available on the market. The majority of manufacturers make breast pumps that require a piston to create a vacuum, causing the nipple to be moved in and out of a barrel at different speeds and intensity. The pump piece, or flange, that goes over the mother's nipple may or may not come in different sizes. This can pose a problem if the mother's nipples are not "standard" size, and as noted earlier, nipple size can change over the course of pumping. Although most women can likely achieve a full milk supply with this type of pump and the correct size flanges, some women find that this type of pump is painful, either because of the flange or the strength of vacuum exerted on the nipple or because they are unable to fully remove available milk from their breast. Although the vacuum can be controlled, it may still be too high for the mother's comfort.

The other type of breast pump, specific only to the Limerick pump at the time of this writing, does not depend on vacuum alone. It combines vacuum and compression, much like that of a suckling baby, to remove breast milk from the breast. The flange comes in one size only and allows for any size nipples to be comfortably compressed instead of pulling them into a tunnel. The vacuum pressures may be decreased more than the other types of pumps but continue to be enough for effective breast milk removal. Often women who are unable to use the vacuum-only type pump because of pain or decreased emptying of the breast find success with this style of pump.

When choosing a brand of pump, the size of the mother's nipples should be taken into account. If using a type of pump that works by moving the nipple in and out of the barrel of a flange, the size of the flange should be determined in accordance with the diameter of the mother's nipple at the *height of expansion* during pumping. This means that just because the nipple starts out being one size at the beginning of the pumping session, it will not necessarily be the same size after 10 or 15 minutes of pumping. In addition, consideration for maternal fluid shifts, as well as differences in individual nipple sizes in the same woman, need to be taken into account.

At all times, the nipple should be centered in the flange and neither the tip nor the shaft of the nipple should be rubbing on the barrel of the flange. Although putting lubricant such as nipple cream on the nipple or on the flange itself might be effective in decreasing nipple discomfort caused by rubbing, it does not adjust for the decreased expansion of the mammary ducts within the too-tight barrel during pumping, which, if not corrected, will lead to a decreased expulsion of breast milk, increased risk for blocked ducts, and decreased long-term milk supply. Ramsay et al. (2006) demonstrated that higher maximum duct diameters were positively related to greater expressed volumes of breast milk. Therefore, a pump that enables interchangeable flange sizes in several increments is ideal when using this piston-type pump (see Photo 17.3).

To view a video of how to properly assess for flange sizing, go to YouTube and watch "Ameda Purely Yours Breast Pump Custom Fit Flange System" (www.youtube.com/watch?v=V1ID5VP65e0).

Hard- and Soft-Rimmed Flanges

Some flanges are supplied as hard rimmed, whereas others come in a soft-rimmed variety. Breasts should ideally conform to the shape of the hard-rimmed flange better than the soft-rimmed ones, just by virtue of shape and

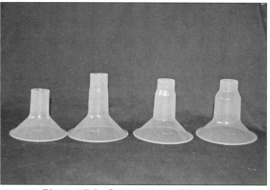

Photo 17.3: Several sizes of flanges.

design, although the soft ones might help create a better seal with some particular breast shapes. Many women state that they find the soft-rimmed flanges more comfortable, but when further investigated, I have found that using the correct size flange is of utmost importance to comfort and that the soft rim of certain flanges decreases the depth of the nipple into the barrel of the flange, thereby decreasing nipple rubbing but being less effective at milk expression. Once switched to a properly fitting hard-rimmed flange, the women all agreed that the new size eliminated the previously felt pain or discomfort associated with the flange that they were using. The Limerick pump not only requires a soft-rimmed flange, but the whole flange itself is made of a soft, pliable silicone, necessary for effective use of this pump.

Vacuum Pressure

Another consideration to be mindful of is the vacuum pressure applied to the nipple during the pumping cycles. Although some women are able to tolerate the preprogrammed vacuum pressure without any discomfort, others may need to adjust the pressure up or down to their own comfort, depending on the elasticity of their nipple/areolar complex. Each pumping session may require different vacuum pressures, depending on the exact placement of the nipple inside the barrel of the flange. A vacuum pressure that is too high can cause damage and cracking at the base of the nipple where it attaches to the areola and therefore should be avoided. Vacuum pressures that can be controlled in very small increments, allowing fine tuning of nipple comfort, is ideal no matter which

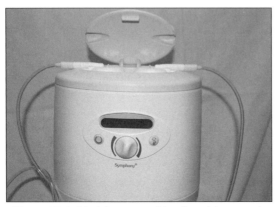

Photo 17.4: Medela pump with adjustable controls for comfort.

type of pump the mother is using (see Photos 17.4 and 17.5). A stronger vacuum does not produce more milk if causing pain or damage to the nipples. Mitoulas, Lai, Gurrin, Larsson, and Hartmann (2002a) concluded that the pressure of the applied vacuum is not related to the volume of expressed breast milk. Milk production and expulsion relies on the comfortable stimulation of the mother's nipple.

CHOOSING THE CORRECT PUMP MODEL

Aside from differing methods of breast milk extraction, several models of breast pumps are available. They range from single manual pumps up through double electric hospital-grade pumps and everything in between. A quick summary of each type of pump and their intended use is given. Keep in mind that for late preterm infants, the Academy of Breastfeeding Medicine (2011) suggests a double electric hospital-grade pump until the maternal milk supply is established and the baby is breastfeeding well without supplementation. Of course, any breast pump is better than no breast pump, and pumping in combination with hand expression is ideal for breast milk removal and increased production.

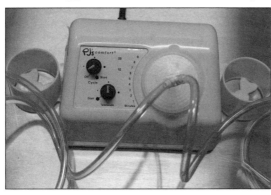

Photo 17.5: Limerick pump with adjustable controls for comfort.

A manual pump is intended for occasional use, designed for mothers who exclusively breastfeed their babies for most feedings and do not need to supplement. The single electric pump was designed for mothers who don't need to pump every day but desire the convenience of an electric pump. The double electric pump is meant for frequent or everyday use, for increasing maternal milk supply, and when there is a need for supplemental feedings (Medela, 2013).

In addition, some double electric pumps have different models, allowing for different patterns of stimulation. As evidenced by studies on vacuum patterns (Kent, Ramsay, Doherty, Larsson, & Hartmann, 2003; Mitoulas et al., 2002b), breast pumps that closely mimic actual infant suckling patterns have greater success with breast milk expression.

Appropriate Flange-to-Breast Contact

Mothers should be instructed not to hold the flanges too tightly to the breast, causing indentation of the breast. This indentation is most noticeable when the mother holds the pump to her breasts by the bottle and not by the actual flange, wears a tight-fitting hands-free bra, or lifts her breasts into the flange before pumping. In most cases, the pump should be placed directly centered over the nipples wherever the breast lies, and held to the breast tightly enough to achieve suction from the pump but not so tight as to indent the breast, because this can cause blockage of milk flow from the area being indented. Blockage of milk flow in any part of the breast can lead to engorgement beyond the blockage, incomplete emptying of the breast, and increased risk for blocked ducts, all of which have a negative effect on maternal comfort, milk supply, and successful breastfeeding.

If the mother is having difficulty holding both flanges to the breast at the same time, she can be taught to cup her breasts with her hands, placing the flange barrel between her index finger and middle finger. This hand placement usually works especially well for women with large breasts or with breasts that may otherwise have difficulty obtaining a seal with the flange. It can decrease the nervousness that mothers experience about the colostrum leaking out from around the edge of the flange by giving her a better feeling of control over flange movement. This positioning works well if the mother has a pillow or two placed vertically behind her, bringing her out from the bed or chair, and allowing more room for her elbows.

Massage During Pumping

Cupping the breast in this way also allows for the mother to massage her breasts during pumping, which has proven to increase milk production, as described earlier (Jones et al., 2001); increases ejection of milk already in the breast, ensuring more complete emptying of the breast (Yokoyama, Ueda, Irahara, & Aono, 1994); and can possibly increase the fat content of the milk (Foda, Kawashima, Nakamura, Kobayashi, & Oku, 2004; Jones et al., 2001). Because late preterm infants often have difficulty with stimulating the mother's milk supply, difficulty maintaining enough stamina to empty the breast, and are in need of extra fat and calories, this technique of massage during pumping should be highly encouraged. More information about breast massage can be found in Chapter 18, "Breast Massage and Hand Expression."

LENGTH OF PUMPING TIMES

Initially, pumping sessions should be limited to 15 to 20 minutes every 2 to 3 hours, until evidence of colostrum or milk flow is seen. Once there is flow, the mother should pump for at least 15 minutes and continue to pump for 2 minutes after the last large drop of breast milk is seen.

As the mother's milk production continues to increase, it is important to continue frequent emptying of the breast to ensure effective milk removal, and longer pumping sessions may be required to empty the breast. As several studies conclude, the regulation of breast milk secretion is dependent on the breast being emptied at each session (Daly & Hartmann, 1995; Jones et al., 2001; Wilde, Prentice, & Peaker, 1995), so proper breast milk expression from the breast is paramount to maintain a proper milk supply. Prime et al. (2012) demonstrated that extending intervals between expressions results in less effective milk removal. Teach the mother that a full breast makes less milk. The American Academy of Breastfeeding Medicine suggests pumping or expressing milk after breastfeeding six to eight times per 24 hours if supplementation is needed, with continued pumping or expressing until the baby is breastfeeding well enough to establish and maintain the mother's milk supply, and recommends the use of a hospital-grade electric pump (Academy of Breastfeeding Medicine, 2011).

If the mother's medical status is unstable after delivery, a nurse or lactation consultant, or perhaps a family member, should pump the mother's breasts for her, encouraging the normal response to nipple stimulation in regard to milk production. Pumping *after* the breastfeeding session or breastfeeding attempt allows the baby to remove whatever colostrum or breast milk he or she can remove and then allows the mother to adequately stimulate her nipples and remove any colostrum or breast milk still available in the breast.

Pumping should be encouraged to continue for as long as supplementation is needed for the baby, then tapered or discontinued to allow for exclusive, uninterrupted breastfeeding and more positive breastfeeding outcomes. If the mother has been pumping and supplementing for an extended period, she has likely become accustomed to knowing how much the baby is actually ingesting, relying on numbers to prove adequate transfer of breast milk. At this point she may need assistance from a lactation consultant to help her become comfortable using other ways to determine the effectiveness of breastfeeding.

SUMMARY

Late preterm infants often are not effective at milk removal from the breast and often need supplemental feeds in the first few days or weeks. Unfortunately, this same period is the most critical time for initiation and establishment of maternal breast milk supply. Without the proper removal of colostrum and breast milk, the attainment of lactogenesis II is prolonged, inhibiting production of a complete milk supply.

To ensure effective milk production as well as make breast milk available for supplementation, the mother of a late preterm infant should start pumping her breasts by 6 hours after delivery and should continue to pump after breastfeeding attempts every 2 to 3 hours for a minimum of 15 minutes, at least during the hospital stay. If the late preterm infant continues to have risk factors for breastfeeding complications, or requires supplementation at the time of discharge, or the mother has risk factors for delayed lactogenesis II, pumping should be encouraged to continue at home until follow-up with a lactation specialist or pediatrician determines that pumping can safely be discontinued.

Proper use of the pump is paramount for continued adherence to use and mothers need to be instructed on correct setup, cleaning, and sizing of pump parts. Pumping should be performed on both breasts simultaneously, even if the baby breastfed from only one breast. With a written plan of the reason for pumping, as well as the milestones needed for the discontinuation of pumping, the mother of the late preterm infant is more likely to have a positive experience and pumping is less likely to have a negative impact on long-term breastfeeding success.

EIGHTEEN

Breast Massage and Hand Expression

EARLY BENEFITS OF HAND EXPRESSION FOR LATE PRETERM INFANTS

Colostrum begins to be made in the breast around 16 weeks gestation and is readily available to the infant immediately after delivery. Although a late preterm infant, who is often sleepy or lethargic after delivery, might not be able to effectively transfer that available colostrum with breastfeeding, hand expression is often helpful to remove the colostrum so it can be given directly to the baby via dropper, syringe, or the mother's finger. Hand expression should be initiated within the first 3 hours of birth and continued at least every 3 hours until the mother's milk supply is in and the baby is feeding well. Colostrum should be given at least every 3 hours regardless of the infant's ability to breastfeed. This ability to feed the baby early, even if the baby is ineffectively latching or suckling, will give him or her needed nutrition, which will decrease the risk for hypoglycemia, dehydration, jaundice, and increased weight loss. Breast massage works complimentary to hand expression to increase blood flow to the breast and enhance breast milk removal.

HAND EXPRESSION: THE RESEARCH BEHIND THE TECHNIQUE

In developing countries, where electric or even manual breast pumps are largely nonexistent, mothers figured out how to hand express their colostrum or breast milk for their babies who were unable to latch or breastfeed directly. Unfortunately, especially in the United States, where equipment and supplies are more readily available, mothers and health care professionals have become reliant on machines to pump breast milk for them. Although the efficacy of electric breast pumps has greatly improved over time, hand expression of colostrum during the first few days after delivery is often much more efficient, and the visible results of accumulating colostrum can greatly boost maternal assurance, especially in unconfident women or women with low self-esteem.

In one study by Slusher et al. (2012), milk volumes from mothers in an African nursery were studied, comparing double electric breast pumps, single nonelectric breast pumps, and hand expression over a 7-day period. These techniques were used by women who were not able to independently breastfeed because of the instability of their baby's status. Although double electric pumps proved to provide the highest mean maternal milk volume, many mothers were able to obtain adequate feeding volumes for their infants using manual breast pumps or manual expression. These findings echoed another study by Slusher et al. (2007), proving hand expression not only to be effective in removing colostrum in the first few days, but effective enough to be used for maintenance of breast milk production in situations where the baby cannot breastfeed directly and there is no other alternative breast pump available.

Morton et al. (2009) studied pump-dependent mothers of preterm infants and observed that after performing mechanical pumping, additional milk could be obtained using hand expression techniques. An 8-week study of 67 new mothers who were taught how to combine hand expression with electric breast pump expression (a technique known as hands-on pumping, or HOP) demonstrated an average milk production between 900 and 1000 mL per day by day 8, compared with typical milk production of 500 to 600 mL average per day using only an electric pump. The researchers determined that expressed milk volumes can be increased by 48% by combining hand expression with mechanical pumping. In addition, mothers who were separated from their infants increased their milk production by 80% when hand expression was used at least six times per day in addition to electric breast pump expression beginning in the first 3 days after delivery (Morton, 2009). This research demonstrates the power of hands-on pumping using both massage and compression during milk expression, which may also play a part when using breast compressions while breastfeeding the late preterm infant. Morton et al. also concluded that it wasn't just the frequency of emptying the breast but the degree of breast emptying that was a significant signal for future milk production.

In another study (Flaherman et al., 2012), researchers performed a randomized trial to compare hand expression with electric breast pump expression. Sixty-eight mothers whose term infants (12–36 hours old) were feeding poorly were followed to determine milk expression volume, maternal nipple pain during expression, and breastfeeding confidence. These women were randomly assigned to either 15 minutes of bilateral electric pumping or 15 minutes of hand expression in the well-baby nursery and postpartum unit. Although the volume range for hand expression was 0 to 5 mL for hand expression and 0 to 40 mL for electric breast pumping, maternal nipple pain and confidence did not differ by intervention. However, at 2 months the mothers assigned to hand expression were more likely still to be breastfeeding than those assigned to the electric pump group (96% vs. 72%). The researchers concluded that hand expression in the early postpartum period appears to improve breastfeeding rates at 2 months compared with electric pump use, and in circumstances where either hand expression or electric pumping would be appropriate for term babies, hand expression should be the method of choice.

Finally, a study done by Ohyama, Watabe, and Hayasaka (2010) was aimed at determining whether pumping using a hospital-grade electric pump was more effective at obtaining maximum amounts of available milk and was more comfortable than hand expression in the first 48 hours after birth. The researchers conducted a sequential cross-over study including 11 women whose babies were admitted to the neonatal intensive care unit (NICU). The women were sequentially allocated to either manually express or use a Medela Symphony breast pump for their first expression after 6 hours following their delivery. They were then to use the other method of expression for the next session, and alternate between methods until seven sessions had been completed for each method, with 3-hour intervals between expressions. The researchers concluded that the mean net milk yield was 2 mL manually and 0.6 mL by mechanical expression. Interestingly, however, more women stated that they experienced "no pain" much more frequently (90% vs. 36%) when using the electric pump than when hand expressing. Perhaps the correct hand expression technique was lacking or taught incorrectly.

From these studies, one can conclude that hand expression of colostrum and breast milk can be very effective for obtaining at least small volumes of nutrition, which is all that is really needed in the first few days of life for late preterm infants. Teaching mothers correct hand expression techniques will minimize or alleviate pain associated with the procedure and increase the effectiveness of breast milk removal.

THE ART OF BREAST MASSAGE: HOW MASSAGE INFLUENCES BREAST MILK FLOW

In an effort to better understand the effects of hands-on breast massage and hand expression of breast milk, a team of health care providers, lactation consultants, and lactating mothers assembled in Russia during three separate occurrences in 2009, 2010, and 2012 (Bolman, Saju, Oganesyan, Kondrashova, & Witt, 2013). Breast massage and hand expression have been popular in Russia since the 1930s, when approximately half the women's population was working and infants were being cared for in daycare centers. Midwives became skilled in hand expression and breast massage techniques to alleviate discomfort and treat complications, and these two techniques still play a vital role in lactation care in Russia to this day. The researchers' aim was to better understand the reasoning and techniques behind the Russians' long tradition of hands-on skills to assist in the resolution of complications of lactation, such as milk stasis, engorgement, and plugged ducts. They concluded that the Russian techniques provide a simple, readily accessible method to encourage mobilization of fluid and to facilitate breast milk removal that can be easily taught to mothers and health care providers.

HAND EXPRESSION TECHNIQUES

Although there is no standard massage technique used throughout Russia, there are common general styles that typically combine massage and hand expression, and all methods are adapted to the patient's breast and specific need, whether that consists of plugged ducts, low milk supply, or engorgement. Both hands are used to massage all around both breasts. Commonly, the breasts are rolled between both hands, or fists are used in a gentle kneading fashion. The massage is performed in a rhythmic motion and can include circular motions, gentle vibrations of the hands, or, in the case of engorgement, placing both hands together around the areola and sliding them toward the base of the breast with or without a gentle rotating motion (also known as reverse pressure softening). Another massage technique, common for plugged ducts, involves placing the fingertips or palms over the affected area and rubbing in quick, repetitive motions back and forth.

Bolman et al. (2013) further describes the basic hand expression technique as follows: "The fingers are positioned on both sides of the nipple… [and then brought gently] together behind the base of the nipple, feeling for a 'stem of tissue fullness,' and moved forward in a rolling motion toward the nipple." Finger placement is then adjusted based on milk flow response.

Jane Morton, pediatrician, clinical professor, and researcher at Stanford University in California, uses a slightly different technique for maximum breast milk removal using hand expression (Morton, 2013a). Her technique eliminates nipple pain, a common complaint in the study by Ohyama et al. (2010), described earlier, because there is no direct pressure on the nipple itself. Early and frequent use of this technique may prove beneficial and essential to the short- and long-term breastfeeding success of late preterm infants. For maximum benefits and results, hand expression should be initiated in the first 3 hours postpartum and performed at least six times every 24 hours.

- Start by washing your hands
- Apply a warm compress over the nipples and breasts for a few minutes, allowing dilation of the ducts
- Perform gentle massage on all areas of both breasts
- Have the mother sit up and lean slightly forward, if she is able to do so
- Form a C with thumb and index finger about an inch back from the areola, with the tip of the thumb and finger in a direct line with the nipple
- Apply steady pressure into the breast and back toward the chest, ensuring you are not just tightening the skin with your fingers
- Compress the thumb and index finger, bringing them together just behind the areola
- Relax the fingers to allow the breast to refill
- Alternate breasts frequently, which simulates the suckling and breathing pauses of a breastfeeding infant
- You may alternate hands on each breast, as well as orientation of fingers on the breasts, decreasing fatigue
- Develop a rhythm similar to a nursing baby

■ It may be helpful to remember *press* (back), *compress* (together), *relax* (fingers) to ensure proper technique

■ It may take a couple of minutes before colostrum flows, just like the initial suckling of the baby while waiting for the milk to let down

■ Perform this technique until colostrum or breast milk is no longer flowing with each compression

Jane Morton's technique can be viewed at http://newborns.stanford.edu/Breastfeeding/HandExpression.html.

Colostrum or breast milk may be collected in a clean container and then fed to the baby using a dropper, syringe, or spoon or by other means if larger amounts of breast milk are being collected this way.

Compared to traditional American hand expression techniques, the hand placement used in Russia is closer to the nipple. In addition, less emphasis is placed on the backward movement toward the chest wall and more focus placed on gentle compression and the rolling motion of the fingers together and forward just behind the nipple base.

HANDS-ON PUMPING

Hands-on pumping, which can increase milk collection volumes and positively affect overall milk supply, requires active maternal participation during electric breast pumping sessions to ensure complete breast drainage. It is easiest performed with a hands-free bra but can be done without one. The following procedure, outlined in Morton's video *Maximizing Milk Procuction and Hands-On Pumping* (2013b), should be followed for maximum results:

■ Massage both breasts

■ Pump both breasts simultaneously

■ Stop pumping once milk flow is reduced to drops

■ Repeat massage

■ Single pump and/or hand express, alternating breasts for several minutes at a time

■ Use the visual sprays of breast milk in the collecting system, as well as any lumps or fullness in the breast, to guide hand usage and positioning

■ Continue until breasts feel empty

With just a little practice, the mother will soon become adept at using a technique that works well for her, enabling her to supply her late preterm infant with extra calories and nutrition needed by her immature baby at this critical time. Even if the late preterm infant appears to be breastfeeding adequately, hand expression and the feeding of the additional colostrum every 2 to 3 hours in the first few days helps ensure adequate intake as well as adequate milk production, both of which will decrease the risk for complications and hospital readmission. Continue hand expression, preferably in combination with mechanical pumping using a double electric breast pump and hands-on pumping, until the baby has proven to be fully competent at breastfeeding and maternal milk supply is fully established.

SUMMARY

Hand expression, breast massage, and hands-on pumping are effective ways to increase milk production, immediately obtain colostrum after a noneffective breastfeeding attempt, and provide extra calories and nutrition to a vulnerable late preterm infant. Using the correct expression technique ensures maximum volume of colostrum with minimal or no nipple discomfort. All mothers of late preterm infants should be taught breast massage and hand expression and encouraged to begin this practice within 3 hours of birth and continue the practice until the baby has proven to breastfeed effectively at all feeds, has passed the period of high risk for complications, and maternal milk supply is greatly increasing. The immediate results of obtaining colostrum can help boost the confidence in an otherwise less than self-confident mother, which is often the case when mothers are faced with the challenges of breastfeeding late preterm infants. Hand expression can also be effective when mechanical breast pumps are not available and the mother is either separated from her baby or the baby is unable to feed directly from the breast.

NINETEEN

Supplemental Feedings

LATE PRETERM INFANT SUPPLEMENTATION DEBATE: WHEN, WHY, HOW MUCH?

In spite of best efforts to breastfeed in the first few weeks, late preterm infants often need more nutrition and calories than can be provided by breastfeeding alone, because of their high metabolic demand, low glucose reserves, increased incidence of jaundice, and weak suckling and delayed maternal lactogenesis II (the dramatic increase in milk supply, or the milk "coming in"). The term *supplementation* refers to giving extra fluids in addition to what the baby receives from breastfeeding alone. Supplementing might be used to increase the amount of fluid intake or to increase the concentration of calories (by adding a fortifier) that the baby receives and can be in the form of the mother's expressed breast milk, pasteurized donor breast milk, breast milk fortified with extra calories, or formula.

Supplementation of extra fluids can be given in several different ways, such as dropper feeding, finger feeding, using a supplemental nursing system or tube and syringe at the breast, spoon feeding, cup feeding and, of course, as most people are familiar with, bottle feeding. In this chapter we explore the controversies involved with supplementation of breastfeeding babies, discuss the most common reasons for needing to supplement late preterm infants, discuss the pros and cons of each method of supplemental feeding, and describe in detail the most effective ways to supplement late preterm infants without disrupting the breastfeeding process.

THE RISKS ASSOCIATED WITH SUPPLEMENTATION

Routine supplementation for breastfeeding babies is contraindicated for several reasons. First, it interferes with the natural breastfeeding process. A baby who receives additional fluids will not feed as frequently or for as long as a hungry baby, decreasing stimulation to the mother's breast, which can delay lactogenesis II and subsequently decrease maternal milk supply.

Second, supplementation of anything other than expressed maternal breast milk (water, glucose water, formula) can significantly alter the pH level of the gut flora, making the gut environment more basic than acidic, which is much more inviting to pathogens. Many studies comparing breast milk feedings with formula feedings and the differences on gut flora, immune responses, and morbidities have been carried out (Carlisle et al., 2013; Donovan et al., 2012; Francavilla et al., 2010; Jacobi & Odle, 2012; Jantscher-Krenn, & Bode, 2012; Li et al., 2012; Palma et al., 2012; Pop, 2012; Poroyko, et al., 2011; Schwartz et al., 2012; Vaarala, 2012; Vester Boler et al., 2013).

Third, supplementation with water or glucose water can cause delayed bilirubin clearance and excess weight loss (American Academy of Pediatrics, 2004; Canadian Paediatric Society, 2007; Dewey, Nommsen-Rivers, Heinig, & Cohen, 2003; Gartner, 2001), leading to longer hospital stays and adverse breastfeeding outcomes.

As Dr. Wight (2012) acknowledges, if formula must be used because of insufficient amounts of the mother's expressed milk or unavailable pasteurized donor breast milk, the next preferred supplemental fluid is protein hydrolysate formulas as opposed to regular infant formula. Hydrolysate formula does not expose the infant to whole cow's milk proteins, reduces bilirubin more rapidly than regular formulas, and, because it is expensive and tastes bad, imparts a message of *temporary* supplementation.

The other risks to consider are the methods of supplementation themselves and how they may affect both short- and long-term breast-feeding outcomes.

SUPPLEMENTATION: THE EXPERTS' OPINIONS

Many experts agree on the potential for late preterm infants needing supplementation, when the benefits often outweigh the risk in this population (Engle, Tomashek, Wallman, & the Committee on the

Fetus and Newborn, 2007; Hubbard, Stellwagen, & Wolf, 2007; Meier, Furman, & Degenhardt, 2007; Walker, 2008; Wang, Dorer, Fleming, & Catlin, 2004; Wight, 2012). Unlike full-term infants, late preterm infants are at risk for excessive weight loss, dehydration, hypoglycemia, and hyperbilirubinemia, all because of their increased rate of metabolism, decreased glucose stores, and decreased bilirubin clearance. Authorities such as the American Academy of Pediatrics (2005) and the Academy of Breastfeeding Medicine (2011) state that supplemental feedings may be necessary when breastfeeding a late preterm infant, as recommended by experts in neonatal and breast-feeding care.

MEDICAL INDICATIONS FOR SUPPLEMENTATION

The Academy of Breastfeeding Medicine (2011) protocol #10 states one of the principles of care as "prevent and promptly recognize frequently encountered problems in breastfed late preterm infants: ...[such as] . . . hypoglycemia . . . hypothermia . . . hyperbilirubinemia . . . dehydration or excessive weight loss . . . [and] failure to thrive," all of which can be caused by insufficient or ineffective breastfeeding, which is commonly exhibited in late preterm infants. The protocol goes on to state the infant should be breastfed or breast milk fed 8 to 12 times in a 24-hour period, that weight loss greater than 3% of birth weight at 24 hours of age or greater than 7% weight loss by day 3 merits further investigation, and that the infant may need supplementation of small quantities of expressed breast milk, donor milk, or formula.

When breastfeeding a late preterm infant, it is important that health care workers and mothers realize that criteria, other than how long the baby appears to be suckling at the breast, needs to be included in the assessment of adequate intake. The baby could, in fact, look to be feeding well, but be ineffective at milk transfer and actually lose weight during each breastfeeding session. In addition, optimal breastfeeding must be encouraged at every breastfeeding attempt, using tools and techniques to increase the success of that particular breastfeeding experience.

Weight loss amounts, diaper assessments, presence of audible swallowing, rate and strength of suckling, signs of dehydration, signs of hypoglycemia, baby's tone, wakefulness, and bilirubin status all need to be incorporated in the assessment of breastfeeding and the decision to start or continue supplementation.

APPROPRIATE SUPPLEMENTATION VOLUME

When supplementing the late preterm infant, we want to be assured the baby is receiving enough nutrition for adequate glucose metabolism, appropriate weight loss in the first few days followed by appropriate weight gain, elimination of excess bilirubin, and for appropriate hydration. We also want to be assured we are giving a small enough amount to encourage frequent breastfeeding attempts, encourage increasing maternal milk supply, and to encourage a positive maternal acceptance to the temporary need for supplementation without interrupting the duration and continuation of breastfeeding.

Although there is limited documentation regarding the amounts with which to supplement a late preterm infant, The Academy of Breastfeeding Medicine (2011) suggests 5 to 10 mL per feeding on day 1, followed by 10 to 30 mL per feeding as needed thereafter. Hubbard et al. (2007) suggest 5 to 10 mL every 2 to 3 hours during the first day of life, followed by 10 to 20 mL every 2 to 3 hours on day 2, and 20 to 30 mL every 2 to 3 hours on day 3. After day 3 the amounts depends on metabolic requirements and feeding tolerance. Wight (2012) suggests slightly lesser amounts in the first couple of days: 2 to 10 mL/feed in the first 24 hours, 5 to 15 mL/feed when 24 to 48 hours old, 15 to 30 mL/feed when 48 to 72 hours old, and 30 to 60 mL/feed when 72 to 96 hours old, when supplementation is medically warranted. Of course, if the mother starts experiencing lactogenesis II and the baby is able to effectively transfer the breast milk, a decrease in the amount of supplementation is encouraged.

METHODS OF SUPPLEMENTATION

Bottles

Probably the most common and well known form of feeding a baby other than breastfeeding is by using a bottle. Much controversy surrounds bottle feeding and its role in causing nipple confusion. Neifert, Lawrence, and Seacat (1995) state that "nipple confusion refers to an infant's difficulty in achieving the correct oral configuration, latching technique, and suckling pattern necessary for successful breast-feeding after bottle feeding or other exposure to an artificial nipple." Although one study supported the idea of nipple confusion (Neifert et al., 1995), others did not find evidence of nipple confusion (Cronenwett et al., 1992) or reported that more research needs to be done in this area for a more accurate assessment (Dowling & Thanattherakul, 2001). Although this conflict between theories continues, one can argue that babies definitely may have a *flow* preference, and in the first few days until the milk production greatly increases, bottle feeding usually results in a more vigorous feeding than breastfeeding does.

Bottle feeding has the advantage of usually being faster to accomplish than breastfeeding, and it is easy to measure the baby's intake, both of which may appeal to new, inexperienced parents and perhaps to health care workers as well. It may also be the least energy-consuming method to feed the really immature (34 week gestation) late preterm infants who are unable to otherwise breastfeed using other devices.

The disadvantages of bottle feeding are numerous, including:

- Decreases the amount of skin-to-skin contact with the mother during feedings, thereby having a negative effect on prolactin levels and milk supply and interfering with thermoregulation of the late preterm baby
- Possibly negatively influences maternal feelings of self-worth because the mother is unable to provide for her baby from the breast
- Increased risk of contamination of bottle parts or of the fluid inside the bottle
- Supplemental fluid may need to be brought to an acceptable temperature for the baby to consume

A study by Howard et al. (2003) demonstrated bottle feeding to have a negative effect on the frequency and duration of breastfeeding. Although other studies (Cronenwett et al., 1992; Schubiger, Schwartz, & Tonz, 1997) attempted to prove or disprove this result, they had several flaws and should be discounted. Cronenwett's results may be dose dependant, and Schubiger et al.'s results were contaminated by many of the control group babies receiving bottles while in the hospital.

Maybe the most important disadvantage of using bottles for late preterm infants is that bottle feeding often decreases physiological stability, resulting in decreased oxygen saturation, increased heart rate, and increased respiratory rate compared with breastfeeding (Goldfield, Richardson, Lee, & Margetts, 2006; Howard et al., 1999; Marinelli, Burke, & Dodd, 2001), indicating the baby's inability to compensate for the increased flow rate. This difficulty in managing the baby's oxygenation and stability during bottle feeding may be lessened by using slow-flow nipples, using paced feeding techniques, and holding the baby in a semi-upright position facing the feeder. Studies by Labbok and Hendershot (1987) and Palmer (1998) both show bottle feeding to increase the risk of malocclusion, leading to a greater chance of the baby needing orthodontic braces later in life.

Although more research needs to be done in the area of bottle feeding and its effect on breastfeeding outcomes, one could definitely argue that if a mother has to attempt to breastfeed, then bottle feed her infant, then pump her breasts to have some breast milk with which to supplement her infant at the next feeding, her resolve to breastfeed could quickly diminish.

Dropper or Syringe

Depending on the amount of supplementation needed, a dropper or syringe can be used to drip expressed breast milk or formula onto the breast just above the baby's lips when he or she is latched. This allows the milk to drip into the baby's mouth as he or she is suckling. Alternately, the dropper can also be inserted into the corner of the baby's mouth before or after breastfeeding, slowly giving needed supplementation, allowing time for licking and swallowing. This method works well in the first day or two when the amount of supplementation is small (5 mL or less) but is time consuming, is often messy, and does not teach the baby proper suckling skills. Periodontal syringes may work well for this method but are expensive and not always available.

Cup Feeding

Several studies of the use, benefit, and safety of cup feeding have been published. Howard et al. (2003) concluded that there were no advantages to cup feeding the general population of healthy breast-fed infants, but it may be beneficial to dyads needing multiple supplements as well as to those who were delivered by cesarean. Lang, Lawrence, and Orme (1994) concluded that infants greater than 30 weeks gestation are able to coordinate swallowing and breathing during cup feeding but might take only small amounts this way initially. Dowling, Meier, DiFiore, Blatz, and Martin (2002) concluded that infants remain physiologically stable during cup feeding but that cup feeding was questionable for efficacy and efficiency. Howard et al. (1999) concluded that cup feeding was similar to bottle feeding in regards to administration times, amounts ingested, and infant physiological stability and took less time than breastfeeding, thereby determining that cup feeding was a good alternative to bottle feeding for supplying supplemental feedings.

Lanese (2011) describes her experience with cup feeding in the neonatal intensive care unit (NICU) she works in as a valuable tool for breastfeeding success that they have employed for more than 22 years, without the danger of nipple confusion. When supplementation is ordered for term infants, they routinely use cup feeding as the method of choice for feeding unless the mother requests bottles. In the preterm population, they found cup feeding to be valuable in the progression from nasogastric tube feedings to full breastfeeding.

One form of cup, known as a *paladai*, is shaped like a gravy boat and is meant to be used to pour small amounts of fluid directly onto the baby's tongue. Aloysius and Hickson (2007) demonstrated increased spillage, increased length of feeding times, and more stress cues with use of the paladai cup in preterm infants. Flint, New, and Davies (2007) concluded that cup feeding cannot be recommended over bottle feeding as a supplement to breastfeeding because it confers no significant benefit in maintaining breastfeeding beyond hospital discharge and carries the unacceptable consequence of a longer stay in hospital.

Whichever form of cup is used, one must be careful to let the baby pace the cup feeding and not pour the milk into the baby's mouth. Cup feeding is likely not an efficient way to supplement a late preterm infant who may need several supplementary feedings.

Spoon Feeding

Spoon feeding is similar to paladai cup feeding, requiring small amounts of colostrum or supplement to be poured into the baby's mouth or onto his or her tongue. Although it might be useful to collect colostrum onto a spoon to feed to the baby, it is time consuming and very difficult to manipulate. The mother has to collect the colostrum from the breast onto the spoon and then transfer the spoon to the baby's mouth without spilling. This method should only be used when the mother has at least one other assistant who can transfer the colostrum to the baby, and perhaps a second assistant to hold the baby in a semi-reclined position for the feeding. It is only practical for very small amounts of supplementation.

Finger Feeding

Finger feeding entails using a small feeding tube connected to a syringe full of expressed breast milk or formula. The person feeding the baby holds the tip of the tubing at the end of his or her index finger and inserts the finger and tubing, finger pad side up, into the baby's mouth and against the roof of the mouth. As the baby suckles, the person feeding the baby slowly pushes the plunger on the syringe to release the milk into the baby's mouth. Although this method usually entices the baby to suckle and ingest the supplemental feeding, care must be taken not to go too fast so as to prevent the baby from choking.

Very little research has been done on the use of finger feeding. Oddy and Glenn (2003) reported on their study in which finger feeding was used with preterm babies while a hospital was changing over to Baby-Friendly status. Although they reported an increase in the number of breastfeeding preterm infants at time of discharge from the special care nursery, they did not determine that the finger feeding caused this increase in breastfeeding rates, as opposed to the Baby-Friendly hospital practices. Until more research into the efficacy and effectiveness of finger feeding is done, finger feeding should be limited to short periods when there are no other alternatives to breastfeeding.

Gavage Feeding

A common feeding method in the NICU is gavage or tube feeding. The tube is placed by a nurse either through the mouth or nose until it reaches the inside of the baby's stomach. Although this might be difficult for a parent to witness, it is the safest and most effective way to feed an infant who is too weak or sick to suck on his or her own. It allows the baby to sleep through feedings if necessary or is used to supplement the baby during or after a breastfeeding session without the expenditure of energy.

Supplemental Nursing System (SNS)

In my opinion, consistent with the opinion of several other experts on late preterm infants (Hubbard et al., 2007; Walker, 2008, 2009), the best way to supplement most late preterm infants is with a #5 French feeding tube and syringe at the breast, especially if supplementation is expected for an extended period (see Photo 19.1). I prefer this setup to the commercial supplemental nursing systems because it is much easier to manage the flow rate, and, unlike a commercial set, this system implies *temporary* supplementation. Although SNSs were initially developed for adoptive breastfeeding (Medela, 2013), many lactation consultants who specialize in late preterm infants are becoming increasingly aware of their benefits for preserv-

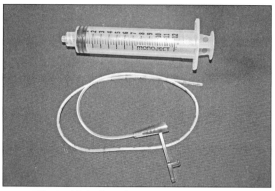

Photo 19.1: Supplemental feeding system consisting of a syringe and feeding tube.

ing breastfeeding for this particular population (Hubbard et al., 2007; Walker, 2008).

An SNS allows the baby to initiate or continue breastfeeding without the interruption of another form of supplementation not at the breast. It enables both breastfeeding and supplementation to be done at the same time, decreasing the time spent to accomplish each feeding. A feeding can easily be consumed within the allotted 20 to 30 minutes (Academy of Breastfeeding Medicine, 2011), and unless the baby latches extremely well, the whole amount of supplementation can be given at one breast, thereby decreasing the amount of energy expenditure of the late preterm baby. The next feeding can be taken from the other breast.

Not only does the SNS decrease the length of time spent on the feeding and supplementation, it increases the efficiency of breast milk removal. Although there is faster and more continuous flow of fluid from the tubing, the baby is likely to stay latched to the breast, increasing the rate and strength of suckling, enhancing the stimulation of the mother's nipple, and transferring not only the supplemental fluid but more of the mother's milk from her breast.

The SNS is the only supplemental feeding method that allows for continued skin-to-skin contact between mother and baby, further boosting the potential for increased maternal milk supply.

Using the SNS decreases the need for "triple feeds," which should increase breastfeeding duration and satisfaction of breastfeeding for the mother. "Triple feeds" refers to the practice of the mother allowing the baby time for breastfeeding attempts, followed by supplementing the baby so that appropriate amounts of nutrition are consumed, followed by pumping her breasts for a minimum of 15 minutes. The triple feeding method, which has generally been the recommendation for mothers who are breastfeeding late preterm infants, is tiresome, frustrating, and impractical. From my own private consulting practice, I have found that mothers who attempt triple feeds for extended periods first drop the breastfeeding attempts, because they are time consuming and often have no visible positive results. They then find their milk supply drops because the baby is no longer at the breast, so often the pumping declines or becomes eliminated, and then the baby is just being bottle fed formula. SNS feedings for late preterm infants help decrease this negative spiral and increase the likelihood of successful exclusive breastfeeding.

The drawbacks to using an SNS to supplement feeds for late preterm infants are minor compared with the benefits. First, the tubing and syringe are not cheap, and extras should be given to the parents in case of loss or damage, so that the mother is never without a set when needed. Second, it may be difficult to feed some 34-week gestation babies or a baby who does not suck strongly enough to transfer milk in this fashion, so another method of supplementation (bottle feeding) might be needed temporarily until the baby matures enough to transfer milk with this method. Third, when used without a nipple shield, the baby might learn to use the tube as a straw, and latch to the tube instead of to the breast. Lastly, it takes dexterity to use the system and time to teach it. However, with a little perseverance and practice, it should become second nature.

PROPER USE OF THE SNS

When using an SNS, the end of the tubing is gently eased into the corner of the baby's mouth and past the gums once the baby has latched to the breast, or placed alongside the nipple just before the baby latches. When placing the tubing into the mouth after latching, care must be taken to avoid touching the baby's cheek and creating a rooting reflex, thereby interrupting the latch. Alternately, the tubing can be placed inside the nipple shield if one is used for latching or suckling purposes.

Tubing placed inside the nipple shield, as opposed to outside the shield, has many added benefits for feeding an infant. The baby is unable to just latch to the tubing, thereby learning to latch appropriately. There can be a reservoir of milk in the nipple shield tip, enticing the baby to suckle before the mother's milk "lets down," enhancing the breastfeeding initiation and maintenance. It is often easier for the mother to manage the tubing, because the application of the nipple shield tethers the tubing to the breast. Advancing the syringe too fast results in leakage from the nipple shield rim instead of choking the infant. Dislodging of the tubing is less likely, keeping the process less messy. Lastly, the tubing can be removed at the end of the supplementation, allowing the baby to continue suckling without disrupting the latch.

The one negative comment I often hear from nurses and lactation consultants who attempt to use the tubing inside the nipple shield is that the tubing does not allow the nipple shield to form a good seal, causing the milk to leak. This only happens if the tubing does not protrude from the *top* of the shield, but comes from the sides or bottom, or if the plunger of the syringe is advanced too quickly or most likely if the nipple shield is incorrectly applied. Please refer to the Chapter 16, "Nipple Shields," for correct application technique.

The plunger should be advanced at a rate that keeps the baby suckling without effort, keeping the reservoir of the nipple shield from becoming empty so the baby does not stop suckling and forget to start again.

If using the tubing *outside* the nipple shield, or alone without a shield, the holes near the end of the tubing must be advanced past the baby's gums. When depressing the plunger on cue with the baby's suckling, if leakage occurs around the baby's lips, the tubing either needs to be advanced slightly or taken out and repositioned. Depressing the plunger should only be done while the baby is suckling, otherwise choking may occur. Mothers may opt to tape the tubing on the areola so the tip of the tubing stays at the end of the mother's nipple. However, this requires extra supplies and some discomfort upon tape removal.

A disadvantage to not using a nipple shield while using the SNS is that there is not a reservoir for the milk to pool in, so it might be difficult to entice the baby to suckle frequently. The benefit to using the tubing without a shield is the baby might possibly form a tight enough seal around the tube and breast to be able to independently depress the plunger, but this is not often the case with late preterm babies who are having difficulties with breastfeeding.

This phenomenon of the infant independently being able to depress the plunger, however, is a good indication that a late preterm baby is able to breastfeed with only minor assistance, possibly ready to decrease amounts or frequency of supplementation if the mother's supply is adequate.

Feeding the baby in a football hold while using the SNS allows for increased maternal arm and hand movement, thereby making this form of supplementation more achievable.

TAPERING SUPPLEMENTATION

Once the late preterm infant starts gaining appropriate weight, is more alert for feeds, is demonstrating adequate urine and stool output, and the risk for high levels of bilirubin decreases, the pediatrician should recommend decreasing or eliminating supplemental feedings. Close assessment of the baby's ability to effectively breastfeed is paramount before discontinuing supplements, making this the ideal time to follow up with a lactation consultant or pediatrician skilled in breastfeeding practices.

Supplementation may be discontinued abruptly if the mother's milk supply is abundant, the baby is very vigorous, and the baby is only consuming a small amount of supplementation because the mother is already supplying most of the feedings by breast. Otherwise, tapering of supplements may be necessary.

Tapering supplementation is usually done by decreasing the frequency or amounts of supplement while *increasing* the frequency and duration of breastfeeding sessions. It is important to note that the baby will likely need to breastfeed more often or for longer durations because the rate of milk flow will likely be less than the previous method of supplementation, and it is important that the baby continues to receive adequate amounts of breast milk. It is also important to discuss with the mother at this time a plan for decreasing frequency of, or cessation of, pumping. Careful follow-up with either the lactation consultant or pediatrician is recommended until the baby proves to be consuming all the feeds by breast without any complications.

SUMMARY

Supplemental feedings for most breastfeeding babies should be avoided unless medically indicated, because there are risks associated with inappropriate supplementation. Late preterm infants often exhibit signs and symptoms warranting supplementation, and health care professionals need to be aware of these issues and initiate supplementation if evaluation and monitoring of breastfeeding manifest suboptimal breastfeeding after appropriate interventions. The method of supplementation should be carefully considered because some methods may create further problems for the breastfeeding mother–baby dyad. Once supplemental feedings have been initiated, a plan should be in place to discontinue the supplementation as soon as medically feasible. With a written plan for the reasons for initiation of supplemental feeds and the milestones needed for discontinuation of supplements, the mother will likely be more cooperative, will feel more in control of her ability to breastfeed her baby, and will work toward the goal of exclusive breastfeeding.

TWENTY

Overcoming Other Challenges

BEYOND JUST BEING LATE PRETERM: OTHER COMPOUNDING FACTORS AFFECTING EFFECTIVE BREASTFEEDING

As if having a late preterm infant is not enough work in itself when it comes to breastfeeding, there are other issues that increase the risks of ineffective breastfeeding. These issues include things such as twins or higher-order multiples, babies who weigh less than 6 pounds at birth, babies with tight frenulums, and maternal nipple size too large for a small baby. Although each of these issues creates difficulties when breastfeeding any baby, late preterm infants face a greater uphill battle in these situations because they are already compromised. Overcoming these challenges often involves the same techniques and procedures already discussed in this book, but may take more time to overcome.

TWINS AND HIGHER-ORDER MULTIPLES

In 2006, multiple pregnancies accounted for 3% of all births in the United States, but there continues to be a disproportionately larger rate of late preterm multiple deliveries than full-term multiple deliveries (Lee, Cleary-Goldman, & D'Alton, 2006). A retrospective case record analysis of 375 cases of multiple pregnancies in Saudi Arabia (Kurdi, Mesleh, Al-Hakeem, Khashoggi, & Khalifa, 2004) was used to analyze the incidence of pregnancies of multiples and the effect on preterm delivery. The overall incidence of twins studied was 14 out of 1,000 births. Premature labor in pregnancies of multiples was seven times greater than in singleton pregnancies (42% vs. 6.4%), and almost half of pregnancies of multiples resulted in delivery by cesarean section.

Sharing the Breast: Twins and Triplets

A mother with late preterm twins or triplets can produce enough breast milk to fully breastfeed her babies, but it takes a lot of vigilance and patience. Pumping and hand expression should be begun as soon as possible to increase readily available colostrum as well as to prime the body for the increased breast milk demand.

Tandem Feeds

It is difficult to do tandem feedings (feeding two babies at the same time), especially with late preterm infants who might not be feeding effectively, but if the mother has someone to help her with feedings, tandem feeding should be encouraged, because often it produces more frequent milk ejection reflexes and more effective feedings from the babies. As one baby suckles, there is a let-down in the other breast, which encourages increased suckling from the second baby, creating further let-downs for the first baby. It is amusing to watch a set of twins breastfeeding at the same time because it looks like they are having a suckling contest.

When breastfeeding babies in tandem, it is often helpful to latch the most difficult baby first. A double breastfeeding pillow is advantageous for positioning babies in the football position. Other positions should not be used for breastfeeding late preterm infants in tandem because the positioning will result in poor latch techniques. Supplementation can be performed during tandem feeding with assistance from another person or by the mother after she becomes comfortable with the technique. If the baby needs supplementation and the mother is unable to perform this task with tandem feeding, single feedings should be done to ensure appropriate ingestion of nutrition.

Feeding in Succession

If twins or triplets are being breastfed one at a time, they should be fed in succession one after the other. If there is prolonged time between each baby's feeding, it will be more difficult to achieve appropriate milk ejections and will increase the energy each baby consumes. It will also become tiring for the mother because the breaks between feedings will be shorter and it will be difficult to find time to pump without interfering with feedings.

Alternate Breasts

Twins should alternate breasts with each feeding, or at least every 24 hours if that is easier for the mother to remember, to ensure appropriate stimulation to each breast, unless there is a medical contraindication, such as one baby has a yeast infection or other infection of the mouth. If feeding triplets, the feeding orders should be altered at each feeding so the third baby is not always receiving an already suckled breast. A good method for this is providing a rotation where the first baby fed at the last feeding becomes the second baby at the next feeding, the second baby at the last feeding will become the third baby at the next feeding, and the third baby fed at the last feeding will become the first baby to feed the next time. The third baby can be offered both breasts each feeding. It takes diligence on the mother's part to ensure effective, timely feedings, so the third baby is not being woken to feed while the first baby already shows signs of hunger.

Supplementation of Twins and Triplets

Marsha Walker (2011) does not advise breastfeeding one or more multiples and supplementing the others at each feeding, or supplementing every baby at each feeding, because this can result in decreased milk production. However, initially with late preterm infants these techniques might be needed in order to ensure appropriate milk intake and until the babies each prove to be effective at breastfeeding. The mother should be encouraged to pump her breasts after feeds every 3 hours to ensure appropriate stimulation for full milk production and to obtain breast milk for supplementation. Once the mother is able to produce a full supply for all her babies and each of the babies is effectively breastfeeding, supplementation should be discontinued to allow for continued full breast milk production and maintenance.

Low Birth Weight, Less Than 6 Pounds

Low-birth-weight or small-for-gestational-age (SGA) late preterm infants are at a greater disadvantage than babies born weighing more than 6 pounds. Hellmeyer et al. (2012) demonstrated that SGA late preterm infants were more often affected by feeding difficulties than their normal-weight late preterm counterparts. Without stored fat for energy consumption, these babies are at greater risk for breastfeeding insufficiency, often because of even more decreased wake cycles than normal late preterm infants and more energy expenditure used during breastfeeding and crying episodes.

Ortigosa Rocha, Bittar, and Zugaib (2010) compared neonatal morbidity and mortality between 50 singleton intrauterine-growth-restricted (IUGR) late preterm infants and 36 singleton appropriate-for-gestational-age (AGA) late preterm infants of comparable gestational ages. IUGR infants were found to be at a higher risk for intraventricular hemorrhage and hypoglycemia. This study reinforces the need for early and frequent feedings, decreased stimuli, appropriate use of nipple shields, and proper positioning, especially with IUGR late preterm infants, to decrease the risk of complications.

Other researchers (Pulver, Guest-Warnick, Stoddard, Byington, & Young, 2009) compared 343,322 newborns born in Utah between 1999 and 2005 to determine how the weight for gestational age affects mortality of late preterm infants. They concluded that late preterm SGA infants were approximately 44 times more likely than term AGA infants to die in their first month and 22 times more likely than AGA term infants to die in their first year of life.

TIGHT FRENULUM

What Is a Tight Frenulum?

A tight frenulum is also known as a short frenulum, short lingual frenulum, tongue tie, and ankyloglossia. Jackson (2012) defines a tongue tie as a lingual frenulum that is short, tight, and restricts normal tongue movement. The tongue-tied baby usually has a mechanical difficulty latching to the breast and maintaining an effective latch. The tight frenulum may be evident at the tip of the tongue or more posteriorly and is classified into four stages.

Significance of a Tight Frenulum

A baby with ankyloglossia can lose excess weight by suckling vigorously, either on just the tip of the mother's nipple or holding onto the breast with his or her lips and attempting suckling deep within the confines of the posterior mouth—neither of which will transfer adequate amounts of colostrum or breast milk. This condition can also cause significant pain and damage to the mother's nipples.

Ongoing Debate Over Treatment for a Tight Frenulum

If a tight frenulum interferes with breastfeeding, it is usually advised by lactation consultants to be surgically corrected. Ankyloglossia is also considered to be a cause of speech difficulties later in life. However, there is much debate between many disciplines (lactation consultants, nurses, physicians, speech pathologists, and elementary teachers) about whether frenotomies really do correct these problems (Messner & Lalakea, 2002; O'Callahan, Macary, & Clemente, 2013; Ostapiuk, 2006; Sethi, Smith, Kortequee, Ward, & Clarke, 2013; Webb, Hao, & Hong, 2013; Wright, 1995). In any case, babies who are unable to latch effectively will show increased weight loss and less effective breast milk transfer and will need assistance with breastfeeding.

How a Tight Frenulum Affects Late Preterm Infant Breastfeeding Success

Late preterm infants often require the use of a nipple shield until breastfeeding is well established. Nipple shields are also commonly used to temporarily resolve breastfeeding issues caused by tight frenulums. Unless the ankyloglossia is obviously causing an issue, using a nipple shield until the late preterm infant is closer to term and better able to prove himself or herself to be effective at breastfeeding is a good strategy to fully appreciate whether or not the frenulum is tight enough to cause breastfeeding difficulties and avoids unnecessary surgical correction in some infants.

NIPPLE/MOUTH SIZE MISMATCH

As many people would suspect, a small baby might have difficulty getting his or her mouth far enough over large nipples to latch effectively. Although this definitely may happen in some cases, often if the baby is positioned appropriately and correct latch techniques are used, there does not seem to be a problem.

If there truly is a size mismatch, steps will need to be taken until the infant is able to latch appropriately. These steps may include using a nipple shield if appropriate or pumping and feeding by a method other than directly at the breast until the baby's mouth is big enough to accommodate the size of his or her mother's nipples.

SUMMARY

Late preterm infants are at risk for several complications related to ineffective breastfeeding. When additional complications to breast-feeding arise, the risk of ineffective breastfeeding and early breastfeed-ing cessation greatly increases. If the mother is unprepared to meet these challenges, either by lack of education regarding the complica-tions or how to overcome these challenges, feelings of frustration and inadequacy may ensue.

TWENTY-ONE

Maternal Satisfaction and Breastfeeding Success: The Big Picture

HEALTH CARE TEAM'S RESPONSIBILITY TO SUPPORT BREASTFEEDING SUCCESS

Ultimately, maternal satisfaction will dictate the success or failure of breastfeeding. Late preterm infants pose breastfeeding challenges unique to their population. Being aware of these challenges and meeting the needs of these infants and their mothers in terms of adequate nutritional intake, appropriate and timely assistance with breastfeeding, correct and consistent instructions for use of breast-feeding tools, and emotional support to the family, who may not be prepared for the challenges associated with breastfeeding a late preterm infant, is essential for successful breastfeeding.

EVIDENCE-BASED RESEARCH DEMONSTRATING SATISFACTION WITH BREASTFEEDING TOOLS

Nipple shields are becoming commonplace in the late preterm breast-feeding population. Although once considered a bad habit, nipple shields have become better suited to meet the needs of the breastfeed-ing late preterm infant. Mothers' satisfaction with using nipple shields for late preterm infants have generally been positive when proper explanations of reasons for use, duration of use, and correct teaching of application techniques have been employed.

Hanna, Wilson, and Norwood (2013) used a longitudinal descrip-tive survey to generate new insights into maternal satisfaction with the use of a nipple shield. The median duration of nipple shield use in their survey group was 6.6 weeks, with close to half the 81 participants stopping nipple shield use by the fifth week postpartum. The majority of mothers in their survey were satisfied with the nipple shield and found it to be helpful, with the vast majority (72%) of responses rated as "extremely helpful."

Although not studying maternal satisfaction of nipple shield use, Meier et al. (2000) found that mothers of late preterm infants and preterm infants used an ultrathin silicone nipple shield for a mean of 32.5 days, which coincided with infants reaching term-corrected age.

Elliott (1996) illustrates how difficult it is for a mother who is struggling with an infant who cannot latch and how quickly a mother's strong desire to breastfeed can be lost if she feels her baby is rejecting her. In this case study, use of a nipple shield was paramount to the baby achieving a proper latch, to maternal satisfaction, and ultimately to breastfeeding success.

Clum and Primomo (1996) describe the transition with premature infants from gavage feeding to breastfeeding as needing the nipple shield as a transitional tool. They state that the nipple shield may also provide the mother with a sense of accomplishment with breastfeeding, leading to a better breastfeeding relationship and thereby contributing to mother and infant health.

In another study (Brigham, 1996), 51 patients used nipple shields for poor latch. Eighty-six percent of respondents reported that use of the ultrathin silicone nipple shield helped them to continue to breastfeed.

Finally, Chertok (2009) performed a prospective, multisite, nonrandomized, between-subject study of 54 mother–infant dyads and concluded that the majority (89.8%) of the mothers reported a positive experience with the nipple shield use and that 67.3% of the mothers reported that the nipple shield helped prevent breastfeeding termination.

EMOTIONAL SATISFACTION FROM BREASTFEEDING LATE PRETERM INFANTS

In an attempt to understand how mothers of late preterm infants manage a multitude of factors affecting their breastfeeding course, Demirci, Happ, Bogen, Albrecht, and Cohen (2012) acknowledged that breastfeeding is more than just a biological phenomenon. They examined 10 late preterm mother–infant dyads over a 6- to 8-week period and found that breastfeeding the late preterm infant was a fluctuating, cascade-like progression of trial and error, influenced by a host of contextual factors and events and culminating with breastfeeding continuation or cessation.

EVIDENCE-BASED CONSISTENT CARE

This study by Demirici et al. describes the need for evidence-based consistent care of late preterm infants to increase their breastfeeding success and maternal satisfaction with breastfeeding. By following the techniques described in this book, the previous rollercoaster effect of poor breastfeeding in the late preterm infant population can be eliminated.

A Canadian study (Mantha, Davies, Moyer, & Crowe, 2008) analyzed data from 74 postpartum women with both high and low self-confidence. Although both groups expressed negative experiences with family-centered maternity care with the same frequency, both groups wanted more nursing support for breastfeeding and postpartum education and teaching. Women whose primary language was neither English or French (the two official Canadian languages) were significantly less confident as new mothers.

TIMELY, CONSISTENT CARE

Timely, consistent, and appropriate care should be given to everyone, but especially to late preterm infants who consistently show ineffective breastfeeding responses. We must be proactive in teaching the family how to care for these special babies, as well as teaching them that these babies are special.

Ekström and Nissen (2006) describe a process-oriented breastfeeding training program for antenatal midwives and postpartum nurses. By including an intervention that guarantees continuity of care, the maternal relationship with her infant and her feelings for her infant were intensified.

Continuity of care is essential for the late preterm infant to effectively breastfeed. Beginning immediately after birth, any unsuccessful breastfeeding attempts can result in a cascade of negative consequences, each having a further negative influence of breastfeeding success. The parents of the late preterm infant must be able to receive appropriate breastfeeding assistance from the health care team and receive consistent, evidence-based education.

COLLABORATIVE CARE FOR IMPROVED BREASTFEEDING OUTCOMES

Although we all want what is best for the mother and baby, our idea of breastfeeding success may be different than the mother's idea of success. Her goals may change as breastfeeding progresses or fails to progress. It is our duty to provide evidence-based information and management strategies to help her attain her breastfeeding goals or reach even further.

Evidence-based information needs to be given by everyone caring for the late preterm mother–infant dyad. Obstetricians and antenatal practitioners should be educating the mother; labor and delivery nurses and postpartum nurses should be using this same approach; and lactation consultants, pediatricians, and everyone else involved in the medical care of this population should be giving the same information. This population of late preterm infants is vulnerable to a multitude of complications, and effective breastfeeding is the key to avoiding or reducing the severity of these complications.

SUMMARY

If a mother of a late preterm infant is well informed about the risks of complications of late preterm infants and the probability of her infant needing some breastfeeding support, she will be better prepared to adapt favorably to the demands of feeding that baby. Consistent teaching and encouragement will help strengthen maternal confidence and ultimately lead to better breastfeeding success. By using the necessary breastfeeding tools and techniques described in this book, late preterm infants will obtain better breastfeeding success rates, will have much fewer breastfeeding-related complications, and will adapt better to their environment and family.

TWENTY-TWO

Putting It All Together: Summary of Important Highlights for Successful Breastfeeding for Late Preterm Infants

LATE PRETERM INFANTS ARE IMMATURE

Late preterm infants are at a high risk of several morbidities because of their undeveloped and immature nervous, respiratory, gastrointestinal, and immune systems. Although they may look just like small versions of full-term babies, they differ greatly in the way they adapt to extra-uterine life, putting them at risk not only for immediate short-term consequences but long-lasting and devastating sequelae.

One of the best ways to overcome these potential health risks is to ensure frequent and effective breastfeeding. Easier said than done! Because of their immaturity, late preterm infants often do not breastfeed well, yet we know that breastfeeding and breast milk feedings are most effective at preventing the complications to which these babies are prone.

ADAPTATION TO EXTRA-UTERINE LIFE IS DIFFERENT FOR LATE PRETERM INFANTS

Within just a couple hours of birth, we know that the late preterm infant's energy stores are likely to be depleted, metabolism is increased to attempt to supply continuous fuel to the brain, and risk for complications such as hypoglycemia, hypothermia, and hyperbilirubinemia are greatly increased. Whereas full-term infants can easily overcome such complications with effective breastfeeding or supplementation, once late preterm infants exhibit these complications, damage to their central nervous system is done, setting them on a different life course, with increased risk for several morbidities, long-term negative consequences, and even death.

Without appropriate and adequate amounts of glucose and nutrition, best obtained from colostrum, late preterm infants will begin their journey through life at a great disadvantage. It is imperative that we change this negative path for these infants. Early, effective breastfeeding is the key to the short-term and long-term health of late preterm infants. Following the techniques described in this book and assisting the mother and baby with breastfeeding will enable the babies to initially obtain adequate amounts of colostrum to maintain homeostasis of all systems and will further ensure an appropriate breast milk supply for continued, effective breastfeeding.

CURRENT EVIDENCE-BASED TECHNIQUES CAN REDUCE FRUSTRATIONS AND COMPLICATIONS

Gone are the days of triple feedings—first trying to breastfeed, taking time to supplement, and then pumping to ensure a supply for the next feeding. Mothers of late preterm infants who have traveled that route have become frustrated, tired, and disappointed, often choosing to give up breastfeeding to keep themselves and their families sane. Feeding a baby using that technique is like a roller coaster ride of emotion, success, failure, and frustration. If supplementation is needed, it should be initiated at the breast within the first few minutes of the feeding. As the late preterm infant matures and requires less supplementation, more vigorous suckling after the supplementation is ingested will be evident.

Evidence-based practice has come a long way from a decade or so ago when the medical profession had just become aware of how late preterm infants differ from both preterm infants and full-term infants. Although these infants continue to be rehospitalized with complications directly related to immaturity and poor breastfeeding, educating everyone about the seriousness of appropriate immediate medical care at birth as well as follow-up and ongoing monitoring of the infant is essential.

SUMMARY OF IMPORTANT BREASTFEEDING STRATEGIES

The main points that are essential to effectively breastfeeding the late preterm infant are summarized next.

Skin-to-Skin Contact and Early, Frequent Feedings

■ Begin skin-to-skin contact immediately after delivery, and continue at least throughout the hospital stay, or longer if effective breast-feeding is not yet established.

■ Ensure that the baby is wearing a cap to decrease heat loss and a diaper to keep the baby dry.

■ Ensure effective sustained suckling at the breast within the first hour of delivery and at least every 3 hours thereafter, using appropriate breastfeeding tools if needed. The baby should be breastfed or receive breast milk or colostrum feeds at least every 3 hours.

Proper Positioning for Breastfeeding

■ Use the football hold for feedings until the baby is more effective at feedings. The football hold is the easiest, safest, and most efficient way to hold the late preterm baby during breastfeeding, ensuring the baby is on his or her side and not supine, and ensuring a latch from the side of, not the front of, the mother's body.

■ Start with making the mother comfortable, stacking two pillows vertically and directly behind her. Usually the closer the pillows are to her bottom, the more comfortable she will be. Not only will the mother be comfortable, but this positioning will allow enough leg room for the infant to be positioned correctly.

■ Position the baby beside the mother, on enough pillows to bring the infant level with the mother's nipple, and turned completely on his or her side with one arm under the mother's breast and one arm above the mother's breast, with hips slightly flexed.

Ensure Proper Latch and Vigorous Suckling

■ Line up the baby's nose with the mother's nipple, not mouth to the nipple. This will ensure appropriate neck and chin extension during the latch.

■ Allow the head to fall back slightly to enable the chin to touch the breast without changing the baby's position. This is best done by supporting the baby between the shoulder blades and guiding the chin in to the breast.

■ Ensure that the baby is brought to the mother's breast and not the breast brought to baby.

■ Instruct the mother not to hold her breast during the latch and feeding unless the breast is very large and the nipple is pointed downward when the breast is at rest. Holding the breast has the risk of improper nipple positioning; movement of the breast once latched can lead to loss of appropriate latch, shallow latch, blocked ducts, and lack of accessibility of hands for performing breast compressions and supplementation.

- Perform the chin-to-breast maneuver to stimulate the baby to attempt to latch. This technique is enough of a stimulus to get a full-term baby to appropriately latch but may not stimulate the late preterm infant to latch because of the immature brain development. If the baby does not attempt to latch with this technique after a couple of tries, without changing the baby's positioning, gently pull down on the baby's chin and wait until the tongue drops before attempting to latch. If the baby still does not latch within one attempt of this technique, a nipple shield is warranted.

Nipple Shield Use May Be Warranted

- Ensure vigorous suckling by performing almost continuous breast compressions, pausing if needed for the infant to swallow. If the baby is not vigorously suckling within a few minutes of latching and breast compressions, a nipple shield is warranted.
- Use a nipple shield if the late preterm infant is not latching, not maintaining the latch for at least 5 minutes the first day of life and greater than 10 minutes every day thereafter, or not vigorously suckling with increased tone.
- Use the appropriate-sized nipple shield, which is usually 24 mm unless the baby is less than 4.5 pounds, then a 20-mm nipple shield may be appropriate. Do not choose nipple shield size based on the size of the mother's nipple because the goal is to get as much breast tissue as possible in the baby's mouth for proper milk transfer and to teach the baby to open the mouth as wide as possible for latching.

Breast Compressions Throughout All Feedings

- Perform breast compressions throughout all feedings until the baby proves to be effective at breastfeeding and the mother's milk supply is fully in.

Double Electric Multiuser Pump

- Use a multiuser double electric breast pump, initiating pumping within 6 hours of birth and continuing to use it 8 to 12 times per 24 hours until the baby is effectively breastfeeding without any further need of supplementation.

Hand Expression

■ Initiate hand expression within 3 hours after birth, or sooner if the baby does not suckle effectively at the initial feeding. Hand expression should then continue to be performed after all breast pumping sessions for 2 to 5 minutes, or longer if colostrum or milk is still flowing.

Colostrum Feedings

■ Feed any expressed colostrum to the baby regardless of the success of the breastfeeding attempt. Dropper feeding works well for small amounts. Colostrum should be available at every feeding.

Supplementation if Medically Warranted

■ Use the appropriate type and amount of breast milk or breast milk substitute if supplementation other than small amounts of colostrum is needed. A feeding tube and syringe is the supplemental nursing system (SNS) method of choice. If using a nipple shield, the feeding tube should be placed inside the nipple shield.

Anticipation of Vulnerability and Needed Assistance

■ Educate the parents about the vulnerability of their late preterm infant.

■ Anticipate that all late preterm infants will need some assistance with breastfeeding. This assistance may be in the form of mechanical pumping and hand expression for the mother, or may include the need for supplemental feedings and nipple shield use for the not-so-immediately-successful infant. Really young or hypotonic late preterm infants (often 34-week-gestation infants) may need to be bottle fed initially if unable to suckle at the breast with an SNS and a nipple shield.

Ongoing Follow-Up

■ Adhere to the pediatrician's follow-up schedule. Ongoing follow-up is necessary until the baby proves to be effective at breastfeeding without any needed supplementation, which often occurs around the baby's original due date. Follow up with a lactation consultant may be warranted throughout the first few weeks. Peer counseling is very helpful for mothers to feel like they are not alone on this journey.

By consistently following the evidence-based practice guidelines discussed in this book, we can greatly increase the rate of breastfeeding success for late preterm infants, thereby decreasing the risk and severity of complications generally associated with the late preterm infant population. The babies will be healthier, the families will be happier, and ideally there will be a mitigation of health care costs associated with late preterm infants.

Late Preterm Infant Breastfeeding Algorithm

See next page.

LATE PRETERM INFANT BREASTFEEDING ALGORITHM

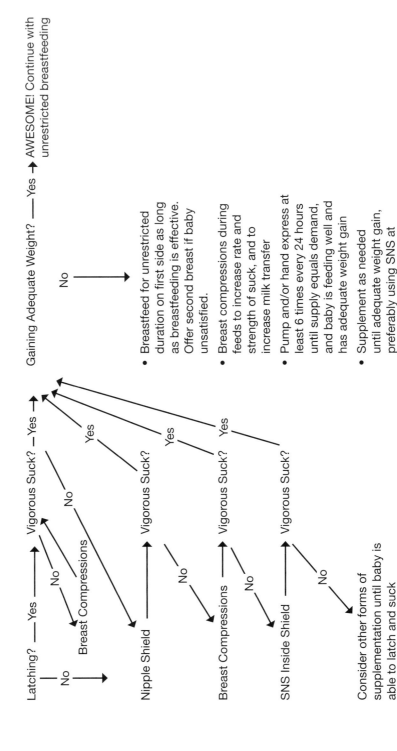

Latching? —— Yes —— Vigorous Suck? — Yes —→ Gaining Adequate Weight? —— Yes —→ AWESOME! Continue with unrestricted breastfeeding

No

No

Breast Compressions

Vigorous Suck?

Yes

Yes

Nipple Shield —→ Vigorous Suck?

No

Breast Compressions —→ Vigorous Suck?

Yes

No

SNS Inside Shield —→ Vigorous Suck?

No

Consider other forms of supplementation until baby is able to latch and suck

No

- Breastfeed for unrestricted duration on first side as long as breastfeeding is effective. Offer second breast if baby unsatisfied.
- Breast compressions during feeds to increase rate and strength of suck, and to increase milk transfer
- Pump and/or hand express at least 6 times every 24 hours until supply equals demand, and baby is feeding well and has adequate weight gain
- Supplement as needed until adequate weight gain, preferably using SNS at breast

Sample In-Hospital Late Preterm Infant Initiative

Reduce Risks of Breastfeeding Difficulties—Health Care Team

- Identify late preterm infants
- Identify maternal risk factors that may affect breastfeeding success
- Provide assistance for at least the first two breastfeeding sessions, and as needed thereafter to ensure frequent breastfeeding of 10 to 12 feedings every 24 hours
  - Babies will often feed well only for the very first feeding then not feed well for a few days
- Maintain nursing staff lactation competences within the scope of nursing practice
- Provide lactation services, ideally with an international board-certified lactation consultant (IBCLC)
- Refer to feeding specialists if feeding difficulties persist
  - Occupational or physical therapist
  - Speech or language pathologists
- Adopt the Baby-Friendly Hospital Initiative's Ten Steps to Successful Breastfeeding

Reduce Risks of Breastfeeding Difficulties—Parent Education

- Explain that the baby is a late preterm infant; define late preterm
- Explain increased risk for ineffective feeding
  - Immature suck, swallow breathe reflexes
  - Decreased milk transfer due to low tone, ineffective suck, decreased stamina
  - Low milk supply due to infrequent nipple stimulation and decreased breast emptying

- Stress the importance of exclusive breastfeeding
  - Value of colostrum
  - Need for frequent, small feedings
- Stress the importance of maintaining skin-to-skin contact whenever possible
  - Improves thermoregulation
  - Improves mothers recognition of early feeding cues
- Teach recognition of early feeding cues
  - Open eyes, head movement, open mouth, tongue thrusting, rooting, suckling fingers or hands
  - Crying is late sign of hunger and uses up energy
- Explain likelihood of having to wake the baby for feedings every 2 to 3 hours
  - Immature brain, excessive sleepiness, does not mean baby is not hungry
- Encourage the mother to ask for breastfeeding assistance
  - Let the staff know immediately if the baby is not feeding well at least every 3 hours
- Provide mother with information about where to obtain breastfeeding help once discharged from the hospital

Assistance With Breastfeeding—Health Care Team

- Assess desire to breastfeed and knowledge or experience with breastfeeding
  - Include mother's experience with breastfeeding late preterm infants
  - If mother's desire is not to breastfeed, support her decision but inform mother of risks of formula feeding
  - Explore reasons for not wanting to breastfeed
  - Explain breastfeeding assistance is available
- Facilitate immediate and uninterrupted skin-to-skin contact for stable infants
- Allow infant time to initiate latch and suckling at first feeding
- Provide assistance for all feedings as needed
- Assure mother's understanding of feeding protocols and need for frequent feedings
- Monitor and document breastfeeding frequency and effectiveness
- A professional with appropriate lactation education and experience should evaluate feedings at least twice every 24 hours
  - Coordination or sucking, breathing, and swallowing
  - Effective latch and milk transfer

- Effective breast compressions during feeds to increase rate and strength of suckling
- Correct positioning of baby
- Comfort of mother, integrity of maternal nipples
- Assess mother's level of fatigue, coping, and ability to effectively breastfeed
- Answer any questions

■ Use of an ultrathin silicone nipple shield if baby unable to latch or does not maintain appropriate suckling after a couple of attempts to latch on own using correct techniques
- Largest size possible should be used to facilitate proper breast-feeding latch and fill buccal cavity

■ Use of a nipple shield requires close follow-up with knowledgeable lactation professional
- Proper weaning techniques should be discussed
- Appropriate use and length of use should be discussed

■ Refer to qualified lactation consultant if available, and/or to feeding specialist if needed

■ Monitor weight at least daily, and more often if excess weight loss is anticipated
- Weight loss of more than 3% per day or 7% to 8% total weight loss by day 3 warrants further investigation and correction (supplement)

■ Assist mother with pumping and hand expression and techniques to feed colostrum to her baby
- Dropper feeding if only a small amount
- Finger feeding if baby unable to latch and suckle
- Supplemental nursing system for larger amounts and for baby who latches well

Assistance With Breastfeeding—Parent Education

■ Review benefits of breastfeeding
- Benefits to both mom and baby

■ Review risks of unnecessary formula or water supplementation
- Decreases frequency of breastfeeding, increases health risk
- Explain that formula supplementation may be warranted if baby not breastfeeding well at least every 3 hours or if there is excessive weight loss
- Encourage frequent expression of colostrum

- Explain the importance of constant skin-to-skin contact
  - Temperature control
  - Early recognition of feeding cues
  - Decreased stress and stimulation
  - Limits exposure to pathogens
- Encourage ongoing skin-to-skin contact while feasible at least until milk supply greatly increases
- Provide verbal and written information about breastfeeding
- Stress the importance of frequent breast feedings, at least 10 to 12 times every 24 hours, watching for cues and waking baby as needed if not awake in 3 hours from beginning of previous feeding
- Stress the importance of correct positioning and ensure mother understands technique
- Stress the importance of breast compressions throughout all feedings until baby is feeding well and milk supply has greatly increased
- Teach appropriate technique for performing breast compressions
- Teach reason for infant needing nipple shield, if appropriate
- Teach correct nipple shield application, use, and care
  - Ensure return application demonstration performed correctly
- Educate about the size of the infant's stomach and the need for small, frequent feedings
- Encourage the mother to ask for assistance when needed and to immediately inform the nurse if unable to wake the baby for feedings or baby does not feed well at least every 3 hours
- Explain the importance of tracking voids and stools
  - To determine adequate intake

Pumping and Hand Expression—Health Care Team
- Provide hospital-grade multiuser pump for use at bedside
- Assist with both hand expression and mechanical pumping within 3 to 6 hours after birth, or sooner if baby unable to transfer colostrum
- All mothers of late preterm infants should begin pumping and hand expression regardless of the infant's ability to breastfeed
  - Increases the chance for a full milk supply
  - Makes colostrum available for supplementation if feeding ability wanes
- Ensure proper flange sizing and appropriate vacuum pressure of pump
- Assess for correct hand expression technique
- Assist with obtaining double electric pump for home use until the baby is term, feeding well, and milk supply is proven to be adequate

Pumping and Hand Expression—Parent Education

- Explain the importance of early and frequent milk expression
  - Late preterm infants tire easily, may not transfer appropriate amounts
  - Frequent removal of colostrum increases milk supply sooner
  - Expressed colostrum available for frequent feeding regardless of infant's ability to breastfeed
- Explain that milk expression is temporary until baby proves himself or herself to be competent at breastfeeding and full milk supply is proven
- Explain complications and incidence of readmissions for late preterm infants and how early and frequent expression will decrease risks
- Teach proper use of pump, sizing of flanges, and appropriate vacuum pressure
  - Size of flanges may require adjusting over time due to fluid shifts
  - Vacuum pressure should never cause pain
- Teach proper hand expression technique
- Teach proper colostrum and breast milk collection, handling, and storage
- Explain importance of complete breast emptying
  - Ensures adequate milk supply
  - Reduces feedback inhibitor of lactation
- Explain need for acquiring hospital grade double electric pump for home use until baby is closer to term, feeding well, and milk supply is adequate
- Explain pumping and hand expression is temporary

Supplementation—Health Care Team

- Supplement only if medically indicated
  - Supplementation of colostrum is medically indicated with late preterm infants
- Supplement with expressed colostrum whenever available
- If further supplementation is needed, the order of preference for supplementation is expressed breast milk, donor human milk, hydrolyzed formula, or formula. Water or glucose water should not be used for supplementation, as it increases health risks
- Supplement small amounts by dropper or larger amounts at the breast by a supplemental nursing system (SNS)

■ If baby is unable to obtain or maintain latch, finger feeding may be required, or bottle feeding if baby is discharged needing this form of supplementation
  • Supplementation at the breast with SNS is the ideal form of supplementation
■ If breastfeeding is inadequate or weight loss greater than acceptable limits, supplement with the following amounts (based on compilation of expert opinion and within confines of Academy of Breastfeeding Medicine protocol) every 2 to 3 hours:
  • First 24 hours: 2 to 10 mL
  • 24 to 48 hours: 5 to 30mL
  • 48 to 72 hours: 15 to 30 mL
  • 72 to 96 hours: 30 to 60mL
■ Evaluate on a daily basis continued need for supplementation
■ Evaluate mother's understanding of feeding plan

Supplementation—Parent Education
■ Explain reason for supplementation
  • Infrequent feedings
  • Ineffective latch
  • Ineffective milk transfer
  • Excessive weight loss
  • Hypoglycemia unrelieved by breastfeeding
  • Increased bilirubin
■ Explain options for supplementing, methods of supplementing, and volumes to be given
■ Stress the value of exclusive breast milk feedings if possible and risks of introducing formula
■ Explain the feeding plan and provide additional written feeding plan
  • Explain that supplementation may be needed until baby is gaining appropriate weight, feeding well, and maternal milk supply is greatly increased
  • Supplementation may be needed until baby has reached intended due date
■ Explain need for follow-up with pediatrician to determine continued supplementation need and breastfeeding efficiency of baby

Follow-Up Care of the Breastfeeding Late Preterm Infant

Follow-up care of the late preterm infant should take a multidisciplinary approach.

A discharge feeding plan should be developed by a lactation consultant, qualified nurse, or feeding specialist before discharge and should be fully understood and able to be adhered to by the parents. All equipment needed to carry out the feeding plan should be acquired before discharge.

The breastfeeding late preterm infant should be seen by the pediatrician or other designated health care provider within 24 to 48 hours of discharge to:

- Determine weight and percent change in weight since birth
- Assess bilirubin clearance
- Assess hydration status
- Review breastfeeding efficiency and need for supplementation
- Assess mother's nipples and breasts for shape, pain, trauma, engorgement, or mastitis (can be done by qualified lactation consultant, if available)

If adjustments to the feeding plan are made, another follow-up visit within 2 to 4 days of adjustment is warranted.

Another follow-up visit with the pediatrician should be made when the infant is 7 days old, which is when bilirubin peaks in late preterm infants.

Weekly weight checks should be continued until the late preterm infant reaches 40 weeks post-conceptual age or until he or she is thriving.

Follow up with a lactation consultant may be required or desired at certain intervals:

- If changes to the feeding plan are necessary
- If the mother is experiencing breast complications
- As baby is weaning off of supplementation or a nipple shield
- When baby first starts fully, exclusively breastfeeding
- Any time a consult is warranted by maternal or infant conditions

Information about how to access outpatient peer support groups should be made available to all breastfeeding mothers.

Sample Patient Teaching Handout: Your Late Preterm Infant

Your baby was born 3 to 6 weeks early (34–36 weeks gestation) and is called a late preterm infant. Being born before term (38–40 weeks gestation) puts your baby at a greater risk for potentially serious health problems. Although your baby may be able to breathe well on his or her own, other problems can arise from being born just a few weeks early.

Parents should be aware that their late preterm infant is at greater risk for breathing problems (respiratory distress). If your baby has any signs of breathing problems, you should immediately inform your nurse or pediatrician or dial 911 once discharged from the hospital.

Your baby is at greater risk for infection. Wash your hands frequently and encourage everyone who comes in contact with your baby to wash their hands often. Limit visitors until your baby is closer to his or her due date. If your baby appears to be sick or has a fever, inform your nurse or pediatrician immediately.

Late preterm infants have less fat than full-term babies and are at greater risk of becoming cold. Keeping your late preterm infant in skin-to-skin contact, especially with the mother, is important to keep the temperature within normal range. Overheating can also be a problem, so avoid overdressing your baby and do not use too many blankets. When not in skin-to-skin contact with the mother, usually your baby will require one more layer of clothing than you are comfortable wearing, and a cap on his or her head. The room temperature does not need to be adjusted for the baby.

Late preterm infants are at greater risk for jaundice, which is when the skin and the white part of the eyes become tinged yellow. Jaundice is a sign of too much bilirubin, which can lead to severe brain damage if the bilirubin climbs to toxic levels. Your baby should be screened for jaundice before discharge from the hospital and should be seen by the pediatrician within 24 to 48 hours after discharge from the hospital if you are breastfeeding. If you notice your baby's skin or the white part of his or her eyes becoming yellow, or if your baby is not feeding well, contact your pediatrician.

Your baby may require smaller, more frequent feedings than a full-term baby would require. It is important to make sure your baby eats well at every feeding. You might need help from a nurse or lactation consultant (breastfeeding specialist) if the baby is not breastfeeding well at least every 2 to 3 hours. Frequent feedings, especially in the first couple of weeks, helps decrease the risk of jaundice and other complications.

Late preterm babies sometimes do not wake up to eat. This does not mean they are not hungry. You must wake your baby and make sure he or she gets fed at least every 3 hours. Undressing the baby and changing his or her diaper will usually wake the baby. Skin-to-skin contact with the mother encourages the baby to wake up more often and breastfeed better.

Breastfeeding is best for both you and your baby. It may be difficult at first to breastfeed your baby, because late preterm infants are often sleepy and unable to latch and suck well. Properly positioning your baby for breastfeeding and helping your baby to latch well will help you and your baby to breastfeed better. Your nurse or lactation consultant will help your baby to breastfeed properly and will show you how to pump your breasts to increase your milk supply. You might need to use some breastfeeding tools for a couple of weeks until your baby becomes mature enough to breastfeed well, and your lactation consultant will help you with these.

Sample Late Preterm Infant Feeding Plan

SKIN TO SKIN

Hold your baby skin to skin as often as possible. Your baby should wear just a diaper and a hat during skin-to-skin contact. Place a blanket loosely over your baby's back or tuck your baby into your gown or clothes.

BREASTFEED

Breastfeed or breast milk feed your baby at least every 3 hours or more often whenever your baby shows feeding cues such as rooting and hand-to-mouth movements or opens eyes. Do not wait for your baby to cry before feeding him or her. If your baby is not waking up at least every 3 hours, you will need to wake him or her by changing the diaper and placing the baby skin to skin.

BREAST COMPRESSIONS

Attempt to breastfeed at least every 3 hours using breast compressions during the feedings to increase the rate and strength of the baby's suckling.

NIPPLE SHIELD

Use the appropriate-sized nipple shield (20 mm or 24 mm) if your baby is not able to latch, does not maintain a latch for at least 5 minutes on the first day or 10 minutes after day 1, or does not suckle strongly.

PUMP AND HAND EXPRESS BOTH BREASTS

Pump both your breasts every 2 to 3 hours, pumping right after a feeding or feeding attempt. Pump both breasts at the same time with a double electric multiuser pump. Initially pump for 15 to 20 minutes, but when your milk supply increases, pump for a minimum of 15 minutes plus an extra 2 minutes after the flow slows down to just a few drops. Hand express both breasts after pumping for about 5 minutes.

COLOSTRUM FEEDINGS

Use the colostrum from pumping and hand expression to feed your baby at the start of the next breastfeeding session if your baby just finished breastfeeding well. If your baby did not breastfeed well, feed that colostrum immediately to your baby using a dropper or supplemental nursing system.

EXTRA (SUPPLEMENTAL) FEEDINGS

If your baby requires more nutrition than you are able to supply initially, supplemental feedings will need to be given until your supply meets your baby's needs. Supplemental feedings should be done at the breast using a tube and syringe (also referred to as a supplemental nursing system [SNS]). Pumping and hand expression are very important to increase your supply.

If colostrum or breast milk is available, use that to feed your baby. Otherwise, donor milk or formula will be needed.

Amounts to be given every 2 to 3 hours if your baby requires extra (supplemental) feedings are as follows:

- First 24 hours: 2 to 10 mL
- 24 to 48 hours old: 5 to 30 mL
- 48 to 72 hours old: 15 to 30 mL
- 72 to 96 hours old: 30 to 60 mL

References

Abrahams, S.W., & Labbok, M.H. (2011). Breastfeeding and otitis media: A review of recent evidence. *Current Allergy and Asthma Reports, 11,* 508–512. doi: 10.1007/s11882-011-0218-3

Academy of Breastfeeding Medicine. (2011). Clinical protocol #10: Breastfeeding the late preterm infant (34 0/7 to 36 6/7 weeks gestation). *Breastfeeding Medicine, 6,* 151–156. First Revision 2011. Retrieved from http://www.bfmed.org. Accessed January 21, 2013. doi: 10.1089/bfm.2011.0990

Adamkin, D.H. (2006). Feeding problems in the late preterm infant. *Clinics in Perinatology, 33,* 831–837.

Adams Waldorf, K.M., & Nelson, J.L. (2008). Autoimmune disease during pregnancy and the microchimerism legacy of pregnancy. *Immunological Investigations, 37,* 631–644. doi: 10.1080/08820130802205886

Aguiar, H., & Silva, A. I. (2011). Breastfeeding: the importance of intervening. *Acta Medica Portuguesa,* 24, 889-896. Epub December 31, 2011.

Aloysius, A., & Hickson, M. (2007). Evaluation of paladai cup feeding in breastfed preterm infants compared with bottle feeding. *Early Human Development, 83,* 619–621.

Alves, J.G., Figueiroa, J.N., Meneses, J., & Alves, G.V. (2012). Breastfeeding protects against type 1 diabetes mellitus: A case-sibling study. *Breastfeeding Medicine, 7,* 25–28. doi: 10.1089/bfm.2011.0009

Amatayakul, K., Vutyavanich, T., Tanthayaphinant, O., Tovanabutra, S., Yutabootr, Y., & Drewett, R.F. (1987). Serum prolactin and cortisol levels after suckling for varying periods of time and the effect of a nipple shield. *Acta Obstetricia et Gynecologica Scandinavica, 66,* 47–51.

Ameda (2013). *The Elite outperforms.* Retrieved from http://www.amedadirect.com/ameda-elite-outperforms-competing-brands. Accessed March 20, 2013.

American Academy of Pediatrics, Committee on Fetus and Newborn. (2011). Postnatal glucose homeostasis in late-preterm and term infants. *Pediatrics, 127,* 575–579. doi: 10.1542/peds.2010-3851

American Academy of Pediatrics, Subcommittee on Hyperbilirubinemia. (2004). Management of hyperbilirubinemia in the newborn infant 35 or more weeks of gestation. *Pediatrics, 114,* 297–316. doi: 10.1542/peds.114.1.297

American Academy of Pediatrics. (2005). Policy statement: Breastfeeding and the use of human milk. *Pediatrics, 115,* 496–506. doi: 10.1542/peds.2004-2491

Andrade, R.A., Coca, K.P., & Abrão, A.C. (2010). Breastfeeding pattern in the first month of life in women submitted to breast reduction and augmentation. *Journal of Pediatrics, 86,* 239–244. doi: 10.2223/JPED.2002

Animated Dissection of Anatomy for Medicine Medical Encyclopedia. (2013). *Placenta abruptio.* Retrieved from http://www.ncbi.nlm.nih.gov/pubmedhealth/PMH0001903. Accessed April 2, 2013.

Arthur, P.G., Smith, M., & Hartmann, P.E. (1989). Milk lactose, citrate, and glucose as markers of lactogenesis in normal and diabetic women. *Journal of Pediatric Gastroenterology and Nutrition, 9,* 488–496.

Auerbach, K.G. (1990). Sequential and simultaneous breast pumping: A comparison. *International Journal of Nursing Studies, 27,* 257–265.

Ayton, J., Hansen, E., Quinn, S., & Nelson, M. (2012). Factors associated with initiation and exclusive breastfeeding at hospital discharge: Late preterm compared to 37 week gestation mother and infant cohort. *International Breastfeeding Journal, 7,* 16. doi: 10.1186/1746-4358-7-16

Baby-Friendly USA. (2011). *The ten steps to successful breastfeeding.* Retrieved from http://www.babyfriendlyusa.org/about-us/baby-friendly-hospital-initiative/the-ten-steps. Accessed January 30, 2013.

Badran, E.F., Abdalgani, M.M., Al-Lawama, M.A., Al-Ammouri, I.A., Basha, A.S., Al Kazaleh, F.A., Saleh, S.S., Al-Katib, F.A., & Khader, Y.S. (2012). Effects of perinatal risk factors on common neonatal respiratory morbidities beyond 36 weeks gestation. *Saudi Medical Journal, 33,* 1317–1323.

Bartick, M., & Reinhold, A. (2010). The burden of suboptimal breastfeeding in the United States: A pediatric cost analysis. *Pediatrics, 125,* e1048–e1056. doi: 10.1542/peds.2009-1616

Baxter, J.K., Sehdev, H.M., & Breckenridge, J.W. (2012). Oligohydramnios imaging. *Medscape Reference.* Retrieved from http://emedicine.medscape.com/article/405914. Accessed April 2, 2013.

Becher, J.C., Bhushan, S.S., & Lyon, A.J. (2012). Unexpected collapse in apparently healthy newborns—a prospective national study of a missing cohort of neonatal deaths and near-death events. *Archives of Disease in Childhood. Fetal and Neonatal Edition, 97,* F30–34. doi: 10.1136/adc.2010.208736

Bell, A.F. White-Traut, R., & Rankin, K. (2012). Fetal exposure to synthetic oxytocin and the relationship with prefeeding cues within one hour postbirth. *Early Human Development, 89,* 137–143. Epub ahead of print, October 16, 2012. doi: 10.1016/j.earlhumdev.2012.09.017

Bérard, A., Le Tiec, M., & De Vera, M.A. (2012). Study of the costs and morbidities of late-preterm birth. *Archives of Disease in Childhood. Fetal and Neonatal Edition, 97,* F329–F334. doi: 10/1136/fetalneonatal-2011-300969

Betzold, C.M., Hoover, K.L., & Snyder, C.L. (2004). Delayed lactogenesis II: A comparison of four cases. *Journal of Midwifery and Women's Health, 49,* 132–137.

Bhutani, V.K., & Johnson, L. (2006). Kernicterus in late preterm infants cared for as term healthy infants. *Seminars in Perinatology, 30,* 89–97.

Blencowe, H., Cousens S., Oestergaard, M.Z., Chou, D., Moller, A.B., Narwal, R., Adler, A., ... & Lawn, J. E. (2012). National, regional, and worldwide estimates of preterm birth rates in the year 2010 with time trends since 1990 for selected countries: A systematic analysis and implications. *Lancet, 379,* 2162–2172. doi:10.1016/S0140-6736(12)60820-4

Blyth, R., et al. (2002). Effect of maternal confidence on breastfeeding duration: an application of breastfeeding self-efficacy theory. *Birth, 29,* 278–284.

Bobrow, K.L., Quigley, M.A., Green, J., Reeves, G.K., & Beral, V. (2012). Persistent effects of women's parity and breastfeeding patterns on their body mass index: Results from the Million Women Study. *International Journal of Obesity.* Epub ahead of print, July 10, 2012. doi: 10.1038/ijo.2012.76

Boccolini, C.S., Boccolini, P.M., de Carvalho, M.L., & de Oliveira, M.I. (2012). Exclusive breastfeeding and diarrhea hospitalization patterns between 1999 and 2008 in Brazilian State Capitals. *Ciencia & Saude Coletiva, 17,* 1857–1863.

Bodley, V., & Powers, D. (1996). Long-term nipple shields use—a positive perspective. *Journal of Human Lactation, 12,* 301–304.

Bolman, M., Saju, L., Oganesyan, K., Kondrashova, T., & Witt, A.M. (2013). Recapturing the art of therapeutic breast massage during breastfeeding. *Journal of Human Lactation.* Epub ahead of print, March 4, 2013. doi:10.1177/0890334413475527

Brigham, M. (1996). Mothers' reports of the outcome of nipple shield use. *Journal of Human Lactation, 12,* 291–297.

Bystrova, K., Widström, A.M., Matthiesen, A.S., Ransjö-Arvidson, A.B., Welles-Nyström, B., Wassberg, C., ... & Uvnäs-Moberg, K. (2003). Skin-to-skin contact may reduce negative consequences of "the stress of being born": A study on temperature in newborn infants, subjected to different ward routines in St. Petersburg. *Acta Paediatrica, 92,* 320–326.

Canadian Paediatric Society, Fetus and Newborn Committee. (2007). Guidelines for detection, management and prevention of hyperbilirubinemia in term and late preterm newborn infants (35 or more weeks' gestation)—summary. *Pediatrics and Child Health, 12,* 401–407.

Capra, L., Tezza, Giovanna, Mazzei, F., & Boner, A.L. (2013). The origins of health and disease: The influence of maternal diseases and lifestyle during gestation. *Italian Journal of Pediatrics, 39,* 7. doi: 10.1185/1824-7288-39-7

Capuco, A.V., Kahl, S., Jack, L.J., Bishop, J.O., & Wallace, H. (1999). Prolactin and growth hormone stimulation of lactation in mice requires thyroid hormones. *Proceedings of the Society for Experimental Biology and Medicine, 221,* 345–351.

Carlisle, E.M., Poroyko, V., Caplan, M.S., Alverdy, J., Morowitz, M.J., & Liu, D. (2013). Murine gut microbiota and transcriptome are diet dependent. *Annals of Surgery, 257,* 287–294. doi: 10.1097/SLA.0b013e318262a6a6

Carolan, M.C., Davey, M.A., Biro, M., & Kealy, M. (2013). Very advanced maternal age and morbidity in Victoria, Australia: A population-based study. *BMC Pregnancy and Childbirth, 13,* 80.

Cedergren, M.I. (2004). Maternal morbid obesity and the risk of adverse pregnancy outcome. *Obstetrics and Gynecology, 103,* 219–224.

Chapman, D.J., Young, S., Ferris, A.M., & Pérez-Escamilla, R. (2001). Impact of breast pumping on lactogenesis stage II after cesarean delivery: A randomized clinical trial. *Pediatrics, 107,* e94. doi: 10.1542/peds.107.6.e94

Charpak, N., Ruiz., J. G., Zupan J, Cattaneo A, Figueroa Z, Tessier R, Cristo M., … Worku, B. (2005). Kangaroo mother care: 25 years after. *Acta Paediatrica, 94,* 514–522.

Chatterton, R.T., Hill, P.D., Aldag, J.C., Hodges, K.R., Belknap, S.M., & Zinaman, M.J. (2000). Relation of plasma oxytocin and prolactin concentrations to milk production in mothers of preterm infants: Influence of stress. *Journal of Clinical Endocrinology & Metabolism, 85,* 3661–3668. doi: 10.1210/jc.85.10.3661

Cheng, Y.W., Kaimal, A.J., Bruckner, T.A., Halloron, D.R., & Caughey, A.B. (2011). Perinatal morbidity. *BJOG: An International Journal of Obstetrics and Gynaecology, 118,* 1446–1454. doi: 10.1111/j.1471-0528.2011.03045.x

Cheong, J.L., & Doyle, L.W. (2012). Increasing rates of prematurity and epidemiology of late preterm birth. *Journal of Pediatrics and Child Health, 48,* 784–788. doi: 10.1111/j.1440-1754.2012.02536.x

Chertok, I.R. (2009). Reexamination of ultra-thin nipple shield use, infant growth and maternal satisfaction. *Journal of Clinical Nursing, 18,* 2949–2955. doi: 10.1111/j.1365-2702.2009.02912

Chertok, I.R., Schneider, J., & Blackburn, S. (2006). A pilot study of maternal and term infant outcomes associated with ultrathin nipple shield use. *Journal of Obstetric, Gynecologic, & Neonatal Nursing, 35,* 265–272.

Chevailier McKechnie, A., & Eglash, A. (2010). Nipple shields: A review of the literature. *Breastfeeding Medicine, 5,* 309–314. doi: 10.1089/bfm.2010.0003

Chouinard-Castonguay, S., Weisnagel, S.J., Tchernof, A., & Robitaille, J. (2013). Relationship between lactation duration and insulin and glucose response among women with prior gestational diabetes. *European Journal of Endocrinology, 168,* 515–523. doi:10.1530/EJE-12-0939

Clapp, D.W. (2006). Developmental regulation of the immune system. *Seminars in Perinatology, 30,* 69–72. doi: 10.1053/j.semperi.2006.02.004

Clum, D., & Primomo, J. (1996). Use of silicone nipple shield with premature infants. *Journal of Human Lactation, 12,* 287–290.

Cohen-Wolkowiez, M., Moran, C., Benjamin, D.K., Cotten, C.M., Clark, R.H., Benjamin Jr., D.K., & Smith, P.B. (2009). Early and late onset sepsis in late preterm infants. *Pediatric Infectious Disease Journal, 28,* 1052–1056.

Colin, A.A., McEvoy, C., & Castile, R.G. (2010). Respiratory morbidity and lung function in preterm infants of 32 to 36 weeks' gestational age. *Pediatrics, 126,* 115–128. doi:10.1542/peds.2009-1381

Collaborative Group on Hormonal Factors in Breast Cancer. (2002). Breast cancer and breastfeeding: Collaborative reanalysis of individual data from 47 epidemiological studies in 30 countries, including 50,302 women with breast cancer and 96,973 women without the disease. *Lancet, 360,* 187–195.

Conde-Agudelo, A., Belizán, J.M., & Diaz-Rossello, J. (2011). Kangaroo mother care to reduce morbidity and mortality in low birthweight infants. *Cochrane*

Database of Systematic Reviews, 16, CD002771. doi: 10.1002/14651858.CD002771. pub2

Consortium on Safe Labor. (2010). Respiratory morbidity in late preterm births. *Journal of the American Medical Association, 304,* 419–425. doi:10.1001/jama.2010.1015

Cronenwett, L., Stukel. T., Kearney, M., Barrett, J., Covington, C., Del Monte, K., … Rippe, L. (1992). Single daily bottle use in the early weeks postpartum and breast-feeding outcomes. *Pediatrics, 90,* 760–766.

Daly, S.E.J., & Hartmann, P.E. (1995). Infant demand and milk supply. part 2: The short-term control of milk synthesis in lactating women. *Journal of Human Lactation, 11,* 27–37. doi: 10.1177/089033449501100120

Daniels, M.C., & Adair, L.S. (2005). Breast-feeding influences cognitive development in Filipino children. *Journal of Nutrition, 135,* 2589–2595.

Darnall, R.A., Ariagno, R.L., & Kinney, H.C. (2006). The late preterm infant and the control of breathing, sleep, and brainstem development: A review. *Clinics in Perinatology, 33,* 883–914.

Davis, E.P., et al. (2011). Children's brain developmental benefits from longer gestation. *Frontiers in Psychology, 2,* 1. Published online February 9, 2011. doi: 10.3389/fpsyg.2011.00001.

Dekker, G.A., Lee, S.Y., North, R.A., McCowan, L.M., Simpson, N.A.B., & Roberts, C.T. (2012). Risk factors for preterm birth in an international prospective cohort of nulliparous women. *PLoS ONE, 7,* e39154. doi: 10.1371/journal.pone.0039154

Delaney, A.L., & Arvedson, J.C. (2008). Development of swallowing and feeding: Prenatal through first year of life. *Developmental Disabilities Research Reviews, 14,* 105–117. doi: 10.1002/ddrr.16

DeLuca, R., Boulvain, M., Irion, O., Berner, M., & Pfister, R.E. (2009). Incidence of early neonatal mortality and morbidity after late-preterm and term cesarean delivery. *Pediatrics, 123,* e1064–1071. doi: 10.1542/peds.2008-2407

Demirci, J.R., Happ, M.B., Bogen, D.L., Albrecht, S.A., & Cohen, S.M. (2012). Weighing worth against uncertain work: The interplay of exhaustion, ambiguity, hope and disappointment in mothers breastfeeding late preterm infants. *Maternal and Child Nutrition.* Epub ahead of print, October1, 2013. doi: 10.1111/j.1740-8709.2012.00463

Derbent, A., Tatli MM, Duran M, Tonbul A, Kafali H, Akyol M, & Turhan, N.O. (2011). Transient tachypnea of the newborn: effects of labor and delivery type in term and preterm pregnancies. *Archives of Gynecology and Obstetrics, 283,* 947–951. doi: 10.1007/s00404-010-1473-6

Dewey, K.G., Nommsen-Rivers, L.A., Heinig, M.J., & Cohen, R.J. (2003). Risk factors for suboptimal infant breastfeeding behavior, delayed onset of lactation, and excess neonatal weight loss. *Pediatrics, 112,* 607–619.

Dey, S.K. (2013). Characteristics of diarrheal illnesses in non-breast fed infants attending a large urban diarrheal disease hospital in Bangladesh. *PLoS One, 8,* e58228. doi: 10.1371/journal.pone.0058228

Do Carmo França-Botelho, A., Ferreira, M.C., França, J.L., França, E.L., & Honório-França, A.C. (2012). Breastfeeding and its relationship with reduction of breast cancer: A review. *Asian Pacific Journal of Cancer Prevention, 13*, 5327–5332.

Dong, Y., & Yu, J.L. (2011). An overview of morbidity, mortality and long-term outcome of late preterm birth. *World Journal of Pediatrics, 7*, 199–204. doi: 10.1007/s12519-011-0290-8

Donovan, S.M., Wang, M., Li, M., Friedberg, I., Schwartz, S.L., & Chapkin, R.S. (2012). Host-microbe interactions in the neonatal intestine: Role of human milk oligosaccharides. *Advances in Nutrition, 3*, 450S–455S. doi: 10.3945/an.112.001859

Dowling, D., & Thanattherakul, W. (2001). Nipple confusion, alternative feeding methods, and breast-feeding supplementation: State of the science. *Newborn and Infant Nursing Reviews, 1*, 7. doi: 10.1053/nbin.2001.28100

Dowling, D.A., Meier, P.P., DiFiore, J.M., Blatz, M., & Martin, R.J. (2002). Cup-feeding for preterm infants: Mechanics and safety. *Journal of Human Lactation, 18*, 13–20.

Dórea, J.G. (2012). Breast-feeding and responses to infant vaccines: Constitutional and environmental factors. *American Journal of Perinatology, 29*, 759–775. doi: 10.1055/s-0032-1316442

Dozier, A.M., Howard, C.R., Brownell, E.A., Wissler, R.N., Glantz, J.C., Ternullo, S.R., … & Lawrence R.A. (2013). Labor epidural anesthesia, obstetric factors and breastfeeding cessation. *Maternal and Child Health Journal, 17*, 689–698. doi: 10.1007/s10995-012-1045-4

Drews, K., & Seremak-Mrozikiewicz, A. (2011). The optimal treatment of thyroid gland function disturbances during pregnancy. *Current Pharmaceutical Biotechnology, 12*, 774–780. doi: 10.2174/138920111795470895

Ekstöm, A., & Nissen, E. (2006). A mother's feelings for her infant are strengthened by excellent breastfeeding counseling and continuity of care. *Pediatrics, 118*, e309–e314. doi: 10.1542/peds.2005-2064

Elliott, C. (1996). Using a silicone nipple shield to assist a baby unable to latch. *Journal of Human Lactation, 12*, 309–313.

Engle, W.A., Tomashek, K.M., Wallman, C., & the Committee on Fetus and Newborn. (2007). "Late-preterm" infants: A population at risk. *Pediatrics, 120*, 1390–1401. doi: 10.1542/peds.2007-2952

Escobar, G.J., Greene, J.D., Hulac, P., Kincannon, E., Bischoff, K., Gardner, M.N., Armstrong, M.A., & France E.K. (2005). Rehospitalization after birth hospitalization: Patterns among infants of all gestation. *Archives of Disease in Childhood, 90*, 125–131.

Feldman, K., Woolcott, C., O'Connell, C., & Jangaard, K. (2012). Neonatal outcomes in spontaneous versus obstetrically indicated late preterm births in a Nova Scotia population. *Journal of Obstetrics and Gynaecology Canada, 34*, 1158–1166.

Fenton, S.E. (2006). Endocrine-disrupting compound and mammary gland development: Early exposure and later life consequences. *Endocrinology, 147*, s18–s24. doi: 10.1210/en.2005-1131

Flaherman, V.J., Gay, B., Scott, C., Avins, A., Lee, K.A., & Newman, T.B. (2012). Randomised trial comparing hand expression with breast pumping for mothers of term infants feeding poorly. *Archives of Disease in Childhood, Fetal and Neonatal Edition, 97,* F18–F23. doi: 10.1136/adc.2010.209213

Flint, A., New, K., & Davies, M.W. (2007). Cup feeding versus other forms of supplemental enteral feeding for newborn infants unable to fully breastfeed. *Cochrane Database of Systematic Reviews, 18,* CD005092.

Foda, M.I., Kawashima, T., Nakamura, S., Kobayashi, M., & Oku, T. (2004). Composition of milk obtained from unmassaged versus massaged breasts of lactating mothers. *Journal of Pediatric Gastroenterology and Nutrition, 38,* 484–487.

Forsling, M.L., Taverne, M.A., Parvizi, N., Elsaesser, F., Smidt, D., & Ellendorff, F. (1979). Plasma oxytocin and steroid concentrations during late pregnancy, partuition and lactation in the miniature pig. *Journal of Endocrinology, 82,* 61–69.

Francavilla, R., Calasso, M., Calace, L., Siragusa, S., Ndagijimana, M., Vernocchi, P., ... & De Angelis, M. (2012). Effect of lactose on gut microbiota and metabolome of infants with cow's milk allergy. *Pediatric Allergy and Immunology, 23,* 420–427. doi: 10.1111/j.1399-3038.2012.01286.x

Gartner, L.M. (2001). Breastfeeding and jaundice. *Journal of Perinatology, 21,* S25–S29.

Geddes, D.T., Kent, J.C., Mitoulas, L.R., & Hartmann, P.E. (2008). Tongue movement and intra-oral vacuum in breastfeeding infants. *Early Human Development, 84,* 471–477. doi: 10.1016/j.earlhumdev.2007.12.008

Geddes, D.T., Sakalidis, V.S., Hepworth, A.R., McClellan, H.L., Kent, J.C., Lai, C.T., & Hartmann, P.E. (2012). Tongue movement and intra-oral vacuum of term infants during breastfeeding and feeding from and experimental teat that released milk under vacuum only. *Early Human Development, 88,* 443–449. doi: 10.1016/j.earlhumdev.2011.10.012

Gizzo, S., Di Gangi, S., Saccardi, C., Patrelli, T.S., Paccagnella, G., Sansone, L., ... Nardelli, G.B. (2012). Epidural analgesia during labor: Impact on delivery outcome, neonatal well-being, and early breastfeeding. *Breastfeeding Medicine, 7,* 262–268. doi: 10.1089/bfm.2011.0099

Goldfield, E.C., Richardson, M.J., Lee, K.G., & Margetts, S. (2006). Coordination of sucking, swallowing, and breathing and oxygen saturation during early infant breast-feeding and bottle-feeding. *Pediatric Research, 60,* 450–455.

Gouyon, J.B., Vintejoux, A., Sagot, P., Burguet, A., Quantin, C., Ferdynus, C., & the Burgundy Perinatal Network. (2010). Neonatal outcome associated with singleton birth at 34–41 weeks of gestation. *International Journal of Epidemiology, 39,* 769–776. doi: 10.1093/ije/dyq037

Hake-Brookes, S.J., & Anderson, G.C. (2008). Kangaroo care and breastfeeding of mother-preterm infant dyads 0-18 months: A randomized, controlled trial. *Neonatal Network, 27,* 151–159.

Hall, R.T., Simon, S., & Smith, M.T. (2000). Readmission of breastfed infants in the first 2 weeks of life. *Journal of Perinatology, 20,* 432–437.

Hanna, S., Wilson, M., & Norwood, S. (2013). A description of breast-feeding outcomes among U.S. mothers using nipple shields. *Midwifery, 29,* 616–621. Epub ahead of print, May 12, 2012. doi: 10.1016/j.midw.2012.05.005

Hapon, M.B., Simoncini, M., Via, G., & Jahn, G.A. (2003). Effect of hypothyroidism on hormone profiles in virgin, pregnant and lactating rats, and on lactation. *Reproduction, 126,* 371–382.

Hartmann, P., & Cregan, M. (2001). Lactogenesis and the effects of insulin-dependent diabetes mellitus and prematurity. *Journal of Nutrition, 131,* 3016S–3020S.

Hauck, F.R., Thompson, J.M., Tanabe, K.O., Moon, R.Y., & Vennemann, M.M. (2011). Breastfeeding and reduced risk of sudden infant death syndrome: Ameta-analysis. *Pediatrics, 128,* 103–110. doi: 10.1542/peds.2010-3000

Hellmeyer, L., Herz, K., Liedtke, B., Wohlmuth, P., Schmidt, S., & Hackeloeer, B.J. (2012). The underestimation of immaturity in late preterm infants. *Archives of Gynecology and Obstetrics, 286,* 619–626. doi: 10.1007/s00404-012-2366-7

Helve, O., Pitkänen, O., Janér, C., & Andersson, S. (2009). Pulmonary fluid balance in the human newborn infant. *Neonatology, 95,* 347–352. doi: 10.1159/000209300

Henly, S.J., Anderson, C.M., Avery, M.D., Hills-Bonczyk, S.G., Potter, S., & Duckett, L.J. (1995). Anemia and insufficient milk in first-time mothers. *Birth, 22,* 86–92.

Herrmann, M., King, K., & Weitzman, M. (2008). Prenatal tobacco smoke and postnatal secondhand smoke exposure and child neurodevelopment. *Current Opinions in Pediatrics, 20,* 184–190. doi: 10.1097/MOP.0b013e3282f56165

Hill, P.D., Aldag, J.C., & Chatterton, R.T. (1996). The effect of sequential and simultaneous breast pumping on milk volume and prolactin levels: A pilot study. *Journal of Human Lactation, 12,* 193–199. doi: 10.1177/089033449601200315

Hoover, K.L., Barbalinardo, L.H., & Platia, M.P. (2002). Delayed lactogenesis II secondary to gestational ovarian theca lutein cysts in two normal singleton pregnancies. *Journal of Human Lactation, 18,* 264–268.

Horwood, L.J., & Fergusson, D.M. (1998). Breastfeeding and later cognitive and academic outcomes. *Pediatrics, 101,* E9.

Howard, C.R., de Blieck, E.A., ten Hoopen, C.B., Howard, F.M., Lanphear, B.P., & Lawrence, R.A. (1999). Physiologic stability of newborns during cup- and bottle-feeding. *Pediatrics, 104,* 1204–1207.

Howard, C.R., Howard, F.M., Lanphear, B., Eberly, S., deBlieck, E.A., Oakes, D., & Lawrence, R.A. (2003). Randomized clinical trial of pacifier use and bottle-feeding or cupfeeding and their effect on breastfeeding. *Pediatrics, 111,* 511–518.

Hubbard, E.T., Stellwagen, L., & Wolf, A. (2007). The late preterm infant: A little baby with big needs (CME). *Contemporary Pediatrics.* Retrieved from http://health.ucsd.edu/women/child/newborn/nicu/spin/staff/Documents/ContemporaryPediatricsThelatepreterminfant_AlittlebabywithbigneedsCME.pdf.

Huddy, C.L., Johnson, A., & Hope, P.L. (2001). Educational and behavioural problems in babies of 32-35 weeks gestation. *Archives of Disease in Childhood. Fetal and Neonatal Edition, 85,* F23–F28.

Hunt, C.E. (2006). Ontogeny of autonomic regulation in late preterm infants born at 34-37 weeks postmenstrual age. *Seminars in Perinatology, 30,* 73–76.

Hüppi, P. S., et al. (1998). Quantitative magnetic resonance imaging of brain development in premature and mature newborns. *Annals of Neurology, 43,* 224–235.

Hurst, N.M. (1996). Lactation after augmentation mammoplasty. *Obstetrics and Gynecology, 87,* 30–34.

Hurst, N.M., Valentine, C.J., Renfro, L., Burns, P. & Ferlic, L. (1997). Skin-to-skin holding in the neonatal intensive care unit influences maternal milk volume. *Journal of Perinatology, 17,* 213–217.

Hygeia. (2013). *EnDeare double breast pump.* Retrieved from hygeiainc.com/shop/double-electric-breast-pumps/endeare-breast-pump

Institute of Medicine (U.S.), Committee on Understanding Premature Birth and Assuring Healthy Outcomes. (2007). Chapter 5. In *Preterm birth: Causes, consequences, and prevention.* Washington, D.C.: National Academies Press. Retrieved from http://www.ncbi.nlm.nih.gov/books/NBK11363. Accessed March 3, 2013.

Institute of Medicine and the Committee on Nutritional Status During Pregnancy and Lactation. (1991). Nutritional status and usual dietary intake of lactating women. In *Nutrition during lactation.* Washington, D.C. The National Academies Press.

Jackson, R. (2012). Improving breastfeeding outcomes: The impact of tongue tie. *Community Practitioner, 85,* 42–44.

Jacobi, S.K., & Odle, J. (2012). Nutritional factors influencing intestinal health of the neonate. *Advances in Nutrition, 3,* 687–696. doi: 10.3945/an.112.002683

James, P.R., & Nelson-Piercy, C. (2004). Management of hypertension before, during, and after pregnancy. *Heart, 90,* 1499-1504.

Jantscher-Krenn, E. & Bode, L. (2012). Human milk oligosaccharides and their potential benefits for the breast-fed neonate. *Minerva Pediatrica, 64,* 83–99.

Jefferies, A.L., and the Canadian Paediatric Society, Fetus and Newborn Committee. (2012). Kangaroo care for the preterm infant and family. *Paediatrics and Child Health, 17,* 141–143.

Johnson, M.J., Petri, M., Witter, F.R., & Repke, J.T. (1995). Evaluation of preterm delivery in a systemic lupus erythematosus pregnancy clinic. *Obstetrics and Gynecology, 86,* 396–399.

Jones, E., Dimmock, P.W., & Spencer, S.A. (2001). A randomized controlled trial to compare methods of milk expression after preterm delivery. *Archives of Disease in Childhood—Fetal and Neonatal Edition, 85,* F91–F95.

Jordan, S.J., Cushing-Haugen, K.L., Wicklund, K.G., Doherty, J.A., & Rossing, M.A. (2012). Breast-feeding and risk of epithelial ovarian cancer. *Cancer Causes & Control, 23,* 919–927. doi: 10.1007/s10552-012-9963-4

Kenny, L.C., (2013). Advanced maternal age and adverse pregnancy outcome: Evidence from a large contemporary cohort. *PLoS One, 8,* e56583. Epub February 20, 2013. doi: 10.1371/journal.pone.0056583

Kent, J.C., Ramsay, D.T., Doherty, D., Larsson, M., & Hartmann, P.E. (2003). Response of breasts to different stimulation patterns of an electric breast pump. *Journal of Human Lactation, 19,* 179–186. doi: 10.1177/0890334403252473

Khashu, M., Narayanan, M., Bhargava, S, & Osiovich, H. (2009). Perinatal outcomes associated with preterm birth at 33 to 36 weeks' gestation: A population-based cohort study. *Pediatrics, 123,* 109–113. doi: 10.1542/peds.2007-3743

Kilicli, F., Dokmetas, H.S., & Acibucu, F. (2013). Sheehan's syndrome. *Gynecological Endocrinology, 29,* 292–295. doi: 10.3109/09513590.2012.752454

Kirkegaard, I., Obel, C., Hedegaard, M., & Henriksen, T.B. (2006). Gestational age and birth weight in relation to school performance of 10-year-old children: A follow-up study of children born after 32 completed weeks. *Pediatrics, 118,* 1600–1606.

Koletzko, B., et al. (2013). Early influences of nutrition on postnatal growth. *Nestlé Nutrition Institute Workshop Series, 71,* 11–27. doi: 10.1159/000342533

Kramer, M.S., et al. (2008). Breastfeeding and child cognitive development: New evidence from a large randomized trial. *Archives of General Psychiatry, 65,* 578–584. doi: 10.1001/archpsyc.65.5.578

Kramer, M.S., & Kakuma, R. (2012). Optimal duration of exclusive breastfeeding. *Cochrane Database of Systematic Reviews, 8,* CD003517, Epub August 15, 2012. doi: 10.1002/14651858.CD003517

Kramer, M.S., Demissie, K., Yang, H., Platt, R.W., Sauvé, R., & Liston, R. (2000). The contribution of mild and moderate preterm birth to infant mortality. Fetal and Infant Health Study Group of the Canadian Perinatal Surveillance System. *Journal of the American Medical Association, 284,* 843–849.

Kurdi, A.M., Mesleh, R.A., Al-Hakeem, M.M., Khashoggi, T.Y., & Khalifa, H.M. (2004). Multiple pregnancy and preterm labor. *Saudi Medical Journal, 25,* 632–637.

Labbok, M.H., & Hendersot, G.E. (1987). Does breast-feeding protect against malocclusion? An analysis of the 1981 Child Health Supplement to the National Health Interview Survey. *American Journal of Preventative Medicine, 3,* 227–232.

Landry, A.M., & Thompson, D.M. (2012). Larygomalacia disease presentation, spectrum, and management. *International Journal of Pediatrics.* Epub ahead of print, February 27, 2012. doi: 10.1155/2012/753526

Lanese, M.G. (2011). Cup feeding—a valuable tool. *Journal of Human Lactation, 27,* 12–13. doi: 10.1177/0890334410396668

Lang, S., Lawrence, C.J., & Orme, R.L'E. (1994). Cup feeding: An alternative method of infant feeding. *Archives of Disease in Childhood, 71,* 365–369.

Larkin, T., Kiehn, T., Murphy, P.K., & Uhryniak, J. (2013). Examining the use and outcomes of a new hospital-grade breast pump in exclusively pumping NICU mothers. *Advances in Neonatal Care, 13,* 75–82. doi: 10.1097/ANC.0b013e31827d4ce3

Larsen, P. D., & Stensaas, S. S. (2003). Pedi neurologic exam: A neurodevelopmental approach. Retrieved from http://library.med.utah.edu/pedineurologicexam/html/dev_anatomy.html#04

Laufer, A.B. (1990). Breastfeeding. Toward resolution of the unsatisfying birth experience. *Journal of Nurse-Midwifery, 35,* 42–45.

Lee, Y.M., Cleary-Goldman, J., & D'Alton, M.E. (2006). The impact of multiple gestations on late preterm (near-term) births. *Clinics in Perinatology, 33,* 777–792.

Leonard, S.A., Labiner-Wolfe, J., Geraghty, S.R., & Rasmussen, K.M. (2011). Associations between high prepregnancy body mass index, breast-milk expression, and breast-milk production and feeding. *American Journal of Clinical Nutrition, 93,* 556–563. doi:10.3945/ajcn.110.002352

Leung, A.K., & Sauve, R.S. (2005). Breast is best for babies. *Journal of the National Medical Association, 97,* 1010–1019.

Li, M., Bauer, L.L., Chen, X., Wang, M., Kuhlenschmidt, T.B., Kuhlenschmidt, M.S., Fahey, G.C. Jr., & Donovan, S.M. (2012). Microbial composition and in vitro fermentation patterns of human milk oligosaccharides and prebiotics differ between formula-fed and sow-reared piglets. *Journal of Nutrition, 142,* 681–690. doi: 10.3945/jn.111.154427

Lim, K.H., Steinberg, G. (2011). Preeclampsia. *Medscape Reference.* Retrieved from http://emedicine.medscape.com/article/1476919. Accessed April 2, 2013.

Limerick, Inc. (2013). *FAQs* (consumer information). Retrieved from http://limerickinc.com Accessed February 27, 2013.

Lindström, K., Winbladh, B., Haglund, B., & Hjern, A. (2007). Preterm infants as young adults: A Swedish national cohort study. *Pediatrics, 120,* 70–77.

Lipkind, H.S., Slopen, M.E., Pfeiffer, M.R., & McVeigh, K.H. (2012). School-age outcomes of late preterm infants in New York City. *American Journal of Obstetrics and Gynecology, 206,* 222.e1–e6. doi: 10.1016/j.ajog.2012.01.007

Lisboa, P.C., Pires, L., de Oliveira, E., Lima, N.S., Bonomo, I.T., Reis, A.M., … & Moura, E.G. (2010). Prolactin inhibition at mid-lactation influences adiposity and thyroid function in adult rats. *Hormone and Metabolic Research, 42,* 562–569. doi: 10.1055/s-0030-1253434

Loftin, R.W., et al. (2010). Late preterm birth. *Reviews in Obstetrics and Gynecology, 3,* 10–19.

Lubow, J.M., How, H.Y., Habli, M., Maxwell, R., & Sibai, B.M. (2009). Indications for delivery and short-term neonatal outcomes in late preterm as compared with term births. *American Journal of Obstetrics and Gynecology, 200,* e30–33. doi:10.1016/j.ajog.2008.09.022

Ma, P., Brewer-Asling, M., & Magnus, J.H. (2013). A case study on the economic impact of optimal breastfeeding. *Maternal and Child Health Journal, 17,* 9–13. doi: 10.1007/s10995-011-0942-2

Ma, X., Huang, C., Lou, S., Lv, Q., Su, W., Tan, J., … & Provincial Collaborative Study Group for Late-Preterm Infants. (2009). The clinical outcomes of late preterm infants: A multi-center survey of Zhejiang, China. *Journal of Perinatal Medicine, 37,* 695–699. doi: 10.1515/JPM.2009.130

Maisels, M.J., & Kring, E. (1998). Length of stay, jaundice, and hospital readmission. *Pediatrics, 101,* 995–998.

Mally, P.V., Hendricks-Muñoz, K.D., & Bailey, S. (2012). Incidence and etiology of late preterm admissions to the neonatal intensive care unit and its associated respiratory morbidities compared to term infants. *American Journal of Perinatology.* Epub ahead of print, October 24, 2012. doi: 10.1055/s-0032-1326989

Mantha, S., Davies, B., Moyer, A., & Crowe, K. (2008). Providing responsive nursing care to new mothers with high and low confidence. *American Journal of Maternal/Child Nursing, 33,* 307–314. doi: 10.1097/01.NMC.0000334899.14592.32

Marasco, L., Marmet, C, & Shell, E. (2000). Polycystic ovary syndrome: A connection to insufficient milk supply? *Journal of Human Lactation, 16,* 143–148.

Marinelli, K.A., Burke, G.S., & Dodd, V.L. (2001). A comparison of the safety of cupfeedings and bottlefeedings in premature infants whose mothers intend to breastfeed. *Journal of Perinatology, 21,* 350–355.

Marsh, R., Gerber, A.J., & Peterson, B.S. (2008). Neuroimaging studies of normal brain development and their relevance for understanding childhood neuropsychiatric disorders. *Journal of the American Academy of Child and Adolescent Psychiatry, 47,* 1233–1251. doi: 10.1097/CHI.0b013e318185e703

Martin, J.A., Hamilton, B.E., Ventura, S.J., Osterman, M.J., Kirmeyer, S., Mathews, T.J., & Wilson, E.C. (2011). Births: Final data for 2009. *National Vital Statistics Reports, 60,* 1–72.

Martin, J.A., Kirmeyer, S., Osterman, M., & Shepherd, R.A. (2009). Born a bit too early: Recent trends in late preterm births. *National Center for Health Statistics Data Brief,* 1–8.

Martin, J.A., Osterman, M.J.K., & Sutton, P.D. (2010). Are preterm births on the decline in the United States? Recent data from the National Vital Statistics System. *National Center for Health Statistics Data Brief, 39,* 1–7.

Martin, R.M., Goodall, S.H., Gunnell, D., & Davey Smith, G. (2007). Breast feeding in infancy and social mobility: 60-year follow-up of the Boyd Orr cohort. *Archives of Disease in Childhood, 92,* 317–321.

Mathur, G.P., Pandey, P. K., Mathur, S., Sharma, S., Agnihotri, M., Bhalla, M., & Bhalla, J.N. (1993). Breastfeeding in babies delivered by cesarean section. *Indian Pediatrics, 30,* 1285–1290.

Matthiesen, A.S., Ransjö-Arvidson, A.B., Nissen, E., & Uvnäs-Moberg,K. (2001). Postpartum maternal oxytocin release by newborns: Effects of infant hand massage and suckling. *Birth, 28,* 13–19. doi: 10.1046/j.1523-536x.2001.00013.x

McCarter Spaulding, D.E., & Kearney, M.H. (2001). Parenting self-efficacy and perception of insufficient breast milk. *Journal of Obstetric, Gynecologic, and Neonatal Nursing, 30,* 515–522.

McCowan, L.M., Dekker, G.A., Chan, E., Stewart, A., Chappell, L.C., Hunter. M., … & SCOPE consortium, et al. (2009). Spontaneous preterm birth and small for gestational age infants in women who stop smoking early in pregnancy: A prospective cohort study. *BMJ, 338,* b1081. doi: 10.1136/bmj.b1081

McDonald, S.W., Benzies, K.M., Gallant, J.E., McNeil, D.A., Dolan, S.M., Tough, S.C. (2012). A comparison between late preterm and term infants on breastfeeding and maternal mental health. *Maternal and Child Health Journal.* Epub ahead of print, October 7, 2012. doi: 10.1007/s10995-012-1153-1

McIntire, D.D., & Leveno, K.J. (2008). Neonatal mortality and morbidity rates in late preterm births compared with births at term. *Obstetrics and Gynecology, 111,* 35–41. doi: 10.1097/01.AOG.0000297311.33046.73

Medela. (2013). *Breastfeeding info, tips and solutions* (consumer information). Retrieved from http://www.medelabreastfeedingus.com/products/category/breast-pumps. Accessed February 27, 2013.

Medela. (2013). *Specialty feeding* (consumer education). Retrieved from medelabreastfeedingus.com/products/51/supplemental-nursing-system-sns. Accessed February 24, 2013.

Medoff Cooper, B., Holditch-Davis, D., Verklan, M.T., Fraser-Askin, D., Lamp, J., Santa-Donato, A., … & Bingham, D. (2012). Newborn clinical outcomes of the AWHONN late preterm infant research-based practice project. *Journal of Obstetric, Gynecologic, and Neonatal Nursing, 41,* 774–785. doi: 10.1111/j.1552-6909.2012.01401.x

Mehta, U.J., Siega-Riz, A.M., Herring, A.H., Adair, L.S., & Bentley, M.E. (2011). Maternal obesity, psychological factors, and breastfeeding initiation. *Breastfeeding Medicine, 6,* 369–376. doi: 10.1089/bfm.2010.0052

Meier, P.P., Brown, L.P., Hurst, N.M., Spatz, D.L., Engstrom, J.L., Borucki, L.C., & Krouse, A.M. (2000). Nipple shields for preterm infants: Effects on milk transfer and duration of breastfeeding. *Journal of Human Lactation, 16,* 106–114.

Meier, P.P., Engstrom, J.l., Janes, J.E., Jegier, B.J., & Loera, F. (2012). Breast pump suction patterns that mimic the human infant during breastfeeding: Greater milk output in less time spent pumping for breast pump-dependent mothers with premature infants. *Journal of Perinatology, 32,* 103–110. doi: 10.1038/jp.2011.64

Meier, P.P., Furman, L.M., & Degenhardt, M. (2007). Increased lactation risk for late preterm infants and mothers: Evidence and management strategies to protect breastfeeding. *Journal of Midwifery and Women's Health, 52,* 579–587.

Melamed, N., Klinger G, Tenenbaum-Gavish K, Herscovici T, Linder N, Hod M, & Yogev Y. (2009). Short-term neonatal outcome in low-risk, spontaneous, singleton, late preterm deliveries. *Obstetrics and Gynecology, 114*(2 Pt 1), 253–260. doi: 10.1097/AOG.0b013e3181af6931

Merriam-Webster's medical desk dictionary. Erythroblastosis fetalis. Retrieved from http://www.merriam-webster.com/medical/erythroblastosis+fetalis. Accessed April 2, 2013.

Messner, A.H., & Lalakea, M.L. (2002). The effect of ankyloglossia on speech in children. *Otolaryngology Head and Neck Surgery, 127,* 539–545.

Milton, C.G. (2010). The Joint Commission's perinatal care measure set overview. *Breastfeeding Medicine, 5,* 257–258.

Mishra, J, & Pati, S. (2004). Importance of thermoregulation in the newborn: Role of brown fat. *Orissa Journal of Medical Biochemistry, 1,* 75–76.

Mitoulas, L.R., Lai, C.T., Gurrin, L.C., Larsson, M., & Hartmann, P.E. (2002). Effect of vacuum profile on breast milk expression using an electric breast pump. *Journal of Human Lactation, 18,* 353–360. doi: 10.1177/089033402237908

Mitra, A.K., Khoury, A.J., Hinton, A.W., & Carothers, C. (2004). Predictors of breastfeeding intention among low-income women. *Maternal Child Health Journal, 8,* 65–70.

Monroy-Torres, R., Naves-Sánchez, J., & Ortega-Garcia, J.A. (2012). Breastfeeding and metabolic indicators in Mexican premature newborns. *Revista de Investigacion Clinica, 64,* 521–528.

Moore, E.R., Anderson, G.C., Bergman, N., & Dowswell, T. (2012,). Early skin-to-skin contact for mothers and their healthy newborn infants. *Cochrane Database of Systematic Reviews,* 5:CD003519 doi:10.1002/14651858.CD003519.pub3

Morales, E., et al. (2012). Effects of prolonged breastfeeding and colostrums fatty acids on allergic manifestations and infections in infancy. *Clinical and Experimental Allergy, 42,* 918–928. doi: 10.1111/j.1365-2222.2012.03969

Morrison, B., Ludington-Hoe, S., & Anderson, G.C. (2006).Interruptions to breastfeeding dyads on postpartum day 1 in a university hospital. *Journal of Obstetric, Gynecologic, and Neonatal Nursing, 35,* 709–716.

Morse, S.B., Zheng, H., Tang, Y., & Roth, J. (2009). Early school-age outcomes of late preterm infants. *Pediatrics, 123,* e622–629. doi: 10.1542/peds.2008-1405

Morton, J. (2013a). *Hand expression of breast milk* (video). Retrieved from http://newborns.stanford.edu/Breastfeeding/HandExpression.html. Accessed March 5, 2013.

Morton, J. (2013b). *Maximizing milk production with hands-on pumping* (video). Retrieved from http://newborns.stanford.edu/Breastfeeding/MaxProduction.html. Accessed March 5, 2013.

Morton, J., Hall, J.Y., Wong, R.J., Thairu, L., Benitz, W.E., & Rhine, W.D. (2009). Combining hand techniques with electric pumping increases milk production in mothers of preterm infants. *Journal of Perinatology, 29,* 757–764. doi:10.1038/jp.2009.87

Mosby's medical and nursing dictionary. (1986). St. Louis, MO: Mosby.

Moster, D., Lie, R.T., & Markestad, T. (2008). Long-term medical and social consequences of preterm birth. *The New England Journal of Medicine, 359,* 262–273. doi:10.1056/NEJMoa0706475

Msolly, A., Gharbi, O., & Ben Ahmed, S. (2013). Impact of menstrual and reproductive factors on breast cancer risk in Tunisia: A case-control study. *Medical Oncology, 30,* 480. doi: 10.1007/s12032-013-0480-4

Muñoz-Quezada, S., et al. (2013). Competitive inhibition of three novel bacteria isolated from faeces of breast milk-fed infants against selected enteropathogens. *The British Journal of Nutrition, 109,* S63–69. doi: 10.1017/S0007114512005600

National Institutes of Health. (2011). *Dietary supplement fact sheet: Vitamin B 12.* Retrieved from http://www.ods.od.nih.gov/factsheets/VitaminB12-Health Professional/#h6. Accessed April 27, 2013.

Neifert, M., Lawrence, R., & Seacat, J. (1995). Nipple confusion: toward a formal definition. *Journal of Pediatrics, 126,* S125–129.

Neville, M.C., & Morton, J. (2001). Physiology and endocrine changes underlying human lactogenesis II. *Journal of Nutrition, 131,* 30055–30085.

Newman, J. (2009). Breastfeeding and jaundice. Retrieved from http://www. breastfeedingonline.com/newman.shtml. Accessed April 16, 2013.

Nicholson, W.L. (1993). The use of nipple shields by breastfeeding women. *Australian College of Midwives Incorporated Journal*, 6, 18–24.

Nkadi, P.O., Merritt, T.A., & Pillers, D.M. (2009). An overview of pulmonary surfactant in the neonate: genetics, metabolism, and the role of surfactant in health and disease. *Molecular Genetics and Metabolism*, 97, 95–101. doi: 10.1016/j.ymgme.2009.01.015

O'Brien, M., Buikstra, E., Fallon, T., & Hegney, D. (2009). Exploring the influence of psychological factors on breastfeeding duration, phase 1: Perceptions of mothers and clinicians. *Journal of Human Lactation*, 25, 55–63. doi: 10.1177/0890334408326071

O'Callahan, C., Macary, S., & Clemente, S. (2013). The effects of office-based frenotomy for anterior and posterior ankyloglossia on breastfeeding. *International Journal of Pediatric Otorhinolaryngology*. Epub ahead of print, March 21, 2013. S0165-5876(13)00082-7. doi: 10.1016/j.ijporl.2013.02.022

Odd, D.E., Emond, A., & Whitelaw, A. (2012). Long-term cognitive outcomes of infants born moderately and late preterm. *Developmental Medicine Child Neurology*, 54, 704–709. doi:10.1111/j.1469-8749.2012.04315.x

Oddy, W.H, & Glenn, K. (2003). Implementing the Baby Friendly Hospital Initiative: The role of finger feeding. *Breastfeeding Review*, 11, 5–10.

Ohyama, M., Watabe, H., & Hayasaka, Y. (2010). Manual expression and electric breast pumping in the first 48 h after delivery. *Pediatrics International*, 52, 39–43. doi: 10.1111/j.1442-200X.2009.02910.x

Oliveira, A.M., Cunha, C.C., Penha-Silva, N., Abdallah, V.O., & Jorge, P.T. (2008). Interference of the blood glucose control in the transition between phases I and II of lactogenesis in patients with type 1 diabetes mellitus. *Arquivos Brasileiros de Endocrinologia e Metabologia*, 52, 473–481.

Ortigosa Rocha, C., Bittar, R.E., & Zugaib, M. (2010). Neonatal outcomes of late-preterm birth associated or not with intrauterine growth restriction. *Obstetrics and Gynecology International*, 2010, 231842. doi: 10.1155/2010/231842

Osborn, L.M., Reiff, M.I., & Bolus, R. (1984). Jaundice in the full-term neonate. *Pediatrics*, 73, 520–525.

Ostapiuk, B. (2006). Tongue mobility in ankyloglossia with regard to articulation. *Annales Academiae Medicae Stetinensis*, 52, 37–47.

Ouyang, D.W., Khairy, P., Fernandes, S.M., Landzberg, M.J., & Economy, K.E. (2010). Obstetric outcomes in pregnant women with congenital heart disease. *International Journal of* Cardiology, *144*, 195–199. doi: 10.1016/j.ijcard.2009.04.006

Padovani, F.H., Duarte, G., Martinez, F.E., & Linhares, M.B. (2011). Perceptions of breastfeeding in mothers of babies born preterm in comparison to mothers of full-term babies. *Spanish Journal of Psychology*, 14, 884–898.

Palma, G.D., Capilla, A., Nova, E., Castillejo, G., Varea, V., Pozo, T., … & Sanz, Y. (2012). Influence of milk-feeding type and genetic risk of developing celiac disease on intestinal microbiota of infants: The PROFICEL study. *PLoS One, 7,* e30791. doi: 10.1371/journal.pone.0030791

Palmer, B. (1998). The influence of breastfeeding on the development of the oral cavity: A commentary. *Journal of Human Lactation, 14,* 93–98.

Papinczak, T.A., & Turner, C.T. (2000). An analysis of personal and social factors influencing initiation and duration of breastfeeding in a large Queensland maternity hospital. *Breastfeeding Reviews, 8,* 25–33.

Park, H.J., Gu, J.H., Jang, J.C., Dhong, E.S., & Yoon, E.S. (2013). Correction of Pectus Excavatum with breast hypoplasia using simultaneous pectus bar procedure and augmentation mammoplasty. *Annals of Plastic Surgery.* Epub ahead of print, March 12, 2013.

Pascal's principle. (2013). In *Encyclopedia Britannica.* Retrieved from http://www.britannica.com/EBchecked/topic/445445/Pascals-principle.

Pop, M. (2012). We are what we eat: How the diet of infants affects their gut microbiome. *Genome Biology, 13,* 152.

Poroyko, V., Morowitz, M., Bell, T., Ulanov, A., Wang, M., Donovan, S., ... & Liu, D.C. (2011). Diet creates metabolic niches in the "immature gut" that shape microbial communities. *Nutricion Hospitalaria, 26,* 1283–1295. doi: 10.1590/S0212-16112011000600015

Porter, M.L., & Dennis, B.L. (2002). Hyperbilirubinemia and the term newborn. *American Family Physician, 65,* 599–607.

Prime, D.K., Kent, J.C., Hepworth, A.R., Trengove, N.J., & Hartmann, P.E. (2012). Dynamics of milk removal during simultaneous breast expression in women. *Breastfeeding Medicine, 7,* 100–106. doi: 10.1089/bfm.2011.0013

Pulver, L.S., Guest-Warnick, G., Stoddard, G.J., Byington, C.L., & Young, P.C. (2009). Weight for gestational age affects the mortality of late preterm infants. *Pediatrics, 123,* e1072–e1077. doi: 10.1542/peds.2008-3288

Radtke, J.V. (2011). The paradox of breastfeeding-associated morbidity among late preterm infants. *Journal of Obstetric, Gynecologic, and Neonatal Nursing, 40,* 9–24. doi: 10.1111/j.1552-6909.2010.01211.x

Raju, T.N. (2012). Developmental physiology of late and moderate prematurity. *Seminars in Fetal and Neonatal Medicine, 17,* 126–131. doi: 10.1016/j.siny.2012.01.010

Raju, T.N.K., Higgins, R.D., Stark, A.R., & Leveno, K.J. (2006). Optimizing care and outcome for late preterm (near-term) infants: A summary of the workshop sponsored by the National Institute of Child Health and Human Development. *Pediatrics, 118,* 1207–1214. doi: 10.1542/peds.2006-0018

Ramachandrappa, A., & Jain, L. (2009). Health issues of the late preterm infant. *Pediatric Clinics of North America, 56,* 565–577. doi: 10.1016/j.pcl.2009.03.009

Ramsay, D.T., Mitoulas, L.R., Kent, J.C., Cregan, M.D., Doherty, D.A., Larsson, M., & Hartmann, P.E. (2006). Milk flow rates can be used to identify and investigate milk ejection in women expressing breast milk using an electric breast pump. *Breastfeeding Medicine, 1,* 14–23.

Rasmussen, K.M., & Kjolhede, C.L. (2004). Prepregnant overweight and obesity diminish the prolactin response to suckling in the first few weeks postpartum. *Pediatrics, 113*, e465–471.

Redstone, F., & West, J.F. (2004).The importance of postural control for feeding. *Pediatric Nursing, 30*, 97–100.

Saigal, S., & Doyle, L.W. (2008). An overview of mortality and sequelae of preterm birth from infancy to adulthood. *Lancet, 371*, 261–269. doi: 10.1016/ S0140-6736(08)60136-1

Sakalidis, V.S., Williams, T.M., Hepworth, A.R., Garbin, C.P., Hartmann, P.E., Paech, M.J., … & Geddes, G.T. (2013). A comparison of early sucking dynamics during breastfeeding after cesarean section and vaginal birth. *Breastfeeding Medicine, 8*, 79–85. doi: 10.1089/bfm.2012.0018

Scher, M.S., Johnson, M.W., Ludington, S.M., & Loparo, K. (2011). Physiologic brain dysmaturity in late preterm infants. *Pediatric Research, 70*, 524–528. doi: 10.1203/PDR.0b013e31822f24af

Schothorst, P.F., Swaab-Barneveld, H., & van Engeland, H. (2007). Psychiatric disorders and MND in non-handicapped preterm children. Prevalence and stability from school into adolescence. *European Child and Adolescent Psychiatry, 16*, 439–448.

Schubiger, G., Schwarz, U., & Tonz, O. (1997). UNICEF/WHO baby-friendly hospital initiative: Does the use of bottles and pacifiers in the neonatal nursery prevent successful breastfeeding? Neonatal Study Group. *European Journal of Pediatrics, 156*, 874–877.

Schwartz, S., Friedberg, I., Ivanov, I.V., Davidson, L.A., Goldsby, J.S., Dahl, D.B., … & Chapkin, R.S. (2012). A metagenomic study of diet-dependent interaction between gut microbiota and host in infants reveals differences in immune response. *Genome Biology, 13*, r32. doi: 10.1186/gb-2012-13-4-r32

Schwarz, E.B., et al. (2009). Duration of lactation and risk factors for maternal cardiovascular disease. *Obstetrics and Gynecology, 113*, 974–982. doi: 10.1097/01. AOG.0000346884.67796.ca

Scott-Pillai, R., Spence, D., Cardwell, C., Hunter, A., & Holmes, V. (2013). The impact of body mass index on maternal and neonatal outcomes: A retrospective study in a UK obstetric population, 2004-2011. *BJOG: An International Journal of Obstetrics and Gynaecology.* Epub ahead of print, March 27, 2013. doi: 10.1111/1471-0528.12193

Sebire, N.J., Jolly, M., Harris, J.P., Wadsworth, J., Joffe, M., Beard. R.W., … & Robinson, S. (2001). Maternal obesity and pregnancy outcome: A study of 287,213 pregnancies in London. *International Journal of Obesity and Related Metabolic Disorders, 25*, 1175–1182.

Sethi, N., Smith, D., Kortequee, S., Ward, V.M., & Clarke, S. (2013). Benefits of frenulotomy in infants with ankyloglossia. *International Journal of Pediatric Otorhinolaryngology.* Epub ahead of print, February 28, 2013. S0165–5876(13)00065–7. doi: 10.1016/j.ijporl.2013.02.005

Shahir, A.K., Briggs, N., Katsoulis, J., & Levidiotis, V. (2013). An observational outcomes study from 1966-2008, examining pregnancy and neonatal outcomes from dialyzed women using data from the ANZDATA registry. *Nephrology, 18,* 276–284. doi: 10.1111/nep.12044

Shapiro-Mendoza, C.K., Tomashek, K.M., Kotelchuck, M., Barfield, W., Nannini, A., Weiss, J., & Declercq, E. (2008). Effect of late-preterm birth and maternal medical conditions on newborn morbidity risk. *Pediatrics, 121,* e223–e232. doi: 10.1542/peds.2006-3629

Shapiro-Mendoza, C.K., Tomashek, K.M., Kotelchuck, M., Barfield, W., Weiss, J., & Evens, S. (2006). Risk factors for neonatal morbidity and mortality among "healthy" late preterm newborns. *Seminars in Perinatology, 30,* 54–60.

Shelton, K.H., Collishaw, S., Rice, F.J., Harold, G.T., & Thapar, A. (2011). Using genetically informative design to examine the relationship between breastfeeding and childhood conduct problems. *European Childhood and Adolescent Psychiatry, 20,* 571–579. doi:10.1007/s00787-011-0224-y

Simonsen, S., Lyon, J.L., Stanford, J.B., Porucznik, C.A., Esplin, M.S., & Varner, M.W. (2013). Risk factors for recurrent preterm birth in multiparous Utah women: A historical cohort study. *BJOG: An International Journal of Obstetrics and Gynaecology.* Epub ahead of print, February 19, 2013. doi: 10.111/1471-0528.12182

Siu, S.C., Sermer. M., Colman, J.M., Alvarez, A.N., Mercier, L.A., Morton, B.C., … & Cardiac Disease in Pregnancy (CARPREG) Investigators. (2001). Prospective multicenter study of pregnancy outcomes in women with heart disease. *Circulation, 104,* 515–521. doi: 10.1161/hc3001.093437

Sloan, S., Gildea, A., Stewart, M., Sneddon, H., & Iwaniec, D. (2008). Early weaning is related to weight and rate of weight gain in infancy. *Child: Care, Health, and Development, 34,* 59–64. doi:10.1111/j.1365-2214.2007.00771.x

Slusher, T. Slusher, I.L., Biomdo, M., Bode-Thomas, F., Curtis, B.A., & Meier, P. (2007). Electric pump use increases maternal milk volume in African nurseries. *Journal of Tropical Pediatrics, 53,* 125–130.

Slusher, T. Slusher, I.L., Keating, E.M., Curtis, B.A., Smith, E.A., Orodriyo, E., … & Nakakeeto, M.K.. (2012). Comparison of maternal milk (breastmilk) expression methods in an African nursery. *Breastfeeding Medicine, 7,* 107–111. doi:10.1089/bfm.2011.0008

Souto, G.C., Giugliani, E.R., Giugliani, C, & Schneider, M.A. (2003). The impact of breast reduction surgery on breastfeeding performance. *Journal of Human Lactation, 19,* 43–49. doi: 10.1177/0890334402239733

Strunk, T. (2012). Responsiveness of human monocytes to the commensal bacterium *Staphylococcus epidermidis* develops late in gestation. *Pediatric Research, 72,* 10–18. doi: 10.1038/pr.2012.48

Su, C.Y., Lin, H.C., Cheng, H.C., Yen, A.M., Chen, Y.H., & Kao, S. (2013). Pregnancy outcomes of anti-hypertensives for women with chronic hypertension: A population-based study. *PLoS One, 8,* e53844. Epub February 6, 2013. doi: 10.1371/journal.pone.0053844

Sugawara, Y. et al. (2013). Lactation pattern and the risk for hormone-related female cancer in Japan: The Ohsaki cohort study. *European Journal of Cancer Prevention, 22,* 187–192. doi: 10.1097/CEJ. 0b013e3283564610

Sunderam, S., Kissin, D.M., Flowers, L., Anderson, J.E., Folger, S.G., Jamieson, D.J., … & Centers for Disease Control and Prevention (CDC). (2012). Assisted reproductive technology surveillance—United States, 2009. *Morbidity and Mortality Weekly Report Surveillance Summaries, 61,* 1–23.

Swamy, G.T., Ostbye, T., & Skjaerven, R. (2008). Association of preterm birth with long-term survival, reproduction, and next-generation preterm birth. *Journal of the American Medical Association, 299,* 1429–1436. doi: 10.1001/jama.299.12.1429

Tomashek, K.M., Shapiro-Mendoza, C.K., Weiss, J., Kotelchuck, M., Barfield, W., Evans, S., Naninni, A., & Declercq, E. (2006). Early discharge among late preterm and term newborns and risk of neonatal morbidity. *Seminars in Perinatology, 30,* 61–68.

Tsai, M.L., Lien R, Chiang MC, Hsu JF, Fu RH, Chu SM, … & Yang, P.H. (2012). Prevalence and morbidity of late preterm infants: Current status in a medical center in northern Taiwan. *Pediatrics and Neonatology, 53,* 171–177. doi: 10.1016/j.pedneo.2012.04.003

Turck, D., et al. (2005). Breast feeding: health benefits for child and mother. *Archives de Pediatrie, 12,* S145–165.

Underwood, M.A., Danielsen, B., & Gilbert, W.M. (2007). Cost, causes and rates of rehospitalization of preterm infants. *Journal of Perinatology, 27,* 614–619.

U.S. Food and Drug Administration (FDA). (2013). *Consumer updates—breast pumps: Don't be misled. Get the* facts. Retrieved from http://www.fda.gov/ForConsumers/ConsumerUpdates/ucm335261.htm. Accessed March 14, 2013.

Vaarala, O. (2012). Is the origin of type 1 diabetes in the gut? *Immunology and Cell Biology, 90,* 271–276. doi: 10.1038/icb.2011.115

Varas, S.M., Jahn, G.A., & Giménez, M.S. (2001). Hyperthyroidism affects lipid metabolism in lactating and suckling rats. *Lipids, 36,* 801–806.

Varas, S.M., Muñoz, E.M., Hapon, M.B., Aguilera Merlo, C.I., Giménez, M.S., & Jahn, G.A. (2002). Hyperthyroidism and production of precocious involution in the mammary glands of lactating rats. *Reproduction, 124,* 691–702.

Verkaln, M.T., & Walden, M. (2010). *Core curriculum for neonatal intensive care nursing* (4th ed.). St. Louis, MO: Saunders Elsevier.

Vester Boler, B.M., Rossoni Serao, M.C., Faber, T.A., Bauer, L.L., Chow, J., Murphy, M.R., & Fahey, G.C. Jr. (2013). In vitro fermentation characteristics of select nondigestible oligosaccharides by infant fecal inocula. *Journal of Agricultural and Food Chemistry*. Epub ahead of print, February 20, 2013.

Vignoles, P., Gire C, Mancini J, Bretelle F, Boubli L, Janky E, Carcopino X.. (2011). Gestational diabetes: A strong independent risk factor for severe neonatal respiratory failure after 34 weeks. *Archives of Gynecology and Obstetrics, 284,* 1099–1104. doi: 10.1007/s00404-010-1810-9

Volpe, J.J. (2009). Brain injury in premature infants: A complex amalgam of destructive and developmental disturbances. *Lancet Neurology, 8,* 110–124. doi: 10.1016/S1474-4422(08)70294-1

Walker, M. (2008). Breastfeeding the late preterm infant. *Journal of Obstetric, Gynecologic, and Neonatal Nursing, 37,* 692–701. doi:10.1111/j.1552-6909.2008. 00293.x

Walker, M. (2009). *Clinics in human lactation. Breastfeeding the late preterm infant. Improving care and outcomes.* Amarillo, TX: Hale Publishing.

Walker, M. (2010). Breastfeeding management for the late preterm infant: Practical interventions for "little imposters." *Clinical Lactation, 1,* 22–26.

Walker, M. (2011). *Breastfeeding management for the clinician: Using the evidence* (2nd ed.). Sudbury, MA: Jones and Bartlett.

Wang, M.L., Dorer, D.J., Fleming, M.P., & Catlin, E.A. (2004). Clinical outcomes of near-term infants. *Pediatrics, 114,* 372–376.

Wang, X., Zuckerman B, Pearson C, Kaufman G, Chen C, Wang G., ... & Xu, X. (2002). Maternal cigarette smoking, metabolic gene morphism, and infant birth weight. *JAMA: The Journal of the American Medical Association, 287,* 195–202.

Wang, Z.X., Luo, D.L., Dai, X., Yu, P., Tao, L., & Li, S.R.. (2012). Polyacrylamide hydrogel injection for augmentation mammaplasty: Loss of ability for breastfeeding. *Annals of Plastic Surgery, 69,* 123–128. doi: 10.1097/SAP. 0b013e318225931c

Watson Genna, C., & Barak, D. (2010). Facilitating autonomous infant hand use during breastfeeding, *Clinical Lactation, 1,* 15–20.

Watson, J., Hodnett, E., Armson, B.A., Davies, B., & Watt-Watson, J. (2012). A randomized controlled trial of the effect of intrapartum intravenous fluid management on breastfed newborn weight loss. *Journal of Obstetric, Gynecologic, and Neonatal Nursing, 41,* 24–32. doi: 10.1111/j.1552-6909.2011.01321.x

Webb, A.N., Hao, W., & Hong, P. (2013). The effect of tongue-tie division on breastfeeding and speech articulation: A systematic review. *International Journal of Pediatric Otorhinolaryngotomy.* Epub ahead of print, March 25, 2013. doi: 10.1016/j.ijporl.2013.03.008

Wight, N.E. (2012). *Clinics in human lactation. Hospital breastfeeding issues. Hypoglycemia, jaundice, and supplementation.* Amarillo, TX: Hale Publishing.

Wiklund, I., Norman, M., Uvnäs-Moberg, K., Ransjö-Arvidson, A.B., & Andolf, E. (2009). Epidural analgesia: Breastfeeding success and related factors. *Midwifery, 25,* e31–38.

Wilde, C.J., Prentice, A., & Peaker, M. (1995). Breast-feeding: Matching supply with demand in human lactation. *Proceedings of the Nutrition Society, 54,* 401–406.

Willis, C.E., & Livingstone, V. (1995). Infant insufficient milk syndrome associated with maternal postpartum hemorrhage. *Journal of Human Lactation, 11,* 123–126.

Wilson-Clay, B. (1996). Clinical use of silicone nipple shields. *Journal of Human Lactation, 12,* 279–285.

Wilson-Clay, B., & Hoover, K. (2005). *The breastfeeding atlas* (3rd ed., pp. 41–45). Manchaca, TX: LactNews Press.

Woods, A.B., Crist, B., Kowalewski, S., Carroll, J., Warren, J., & Robertson, J. (2012). A cross-sectional analysis of the effect of patient-controlled epidural analgesia versus patient controlled analgesia on postcesarean pain and breast-feeding. *Journal of Obstetric, Gynecologic, and Neonatal Nursing, 41,* 339–346. doi: 10.1111/j.1552-6909.2012.01370.x

Woolridge, M.W., Baum, J.D., & Drewett, R.F. (1980).Effect of a traditional and of a new nipple shield on suckling patterns and milk flow. *Early Human Development, 4,* 357–364.

World Health Organization. (1981). *International code of marketing of breast-milk substitutes.* Geneva, Switzerland: WHO. Retrieved from http://www.who.int/nutrition/publications/code_english.pdf. Accessed January 30, 2013.

World Health Organization (2012). *World Prematurity Day highlights effective, low-cost care.* Geneva, Switzerland: WHO. Retrieved from http://www.who.int/maternal_child_adolescent/news_events/news/2012/world_prematurity_day/en/. Accessed March 6, 2013.

World Health Organization. (2013). *BMI classification.* Geneva, Switzerland: WHO. Retrieved from http://apps.who.int/bmi/index.jsp. Accessed April 4, 2013.

Wright, J.E. (1995). Tongue-tie. *Journal of Paediatrics and Child Health, 31,* 276–278.

Xie, M., Zhang, C., Wang, J.L., Wang, S.M., & Zhang, X.H. (2012). Analysis of the perinatal outcome and risk factors for pregnancies complicated with chronic renal diseases. *Zhonghua Fu Chan Ke Za Zhi, 47,* 161–165.

Yamauchi, Y., & Yamanouchi, I. (1990). Breast-feeding frequency during the first 24 hours after birth in full-term neonates. *Pediatrics, 86,* 171–175.

Yanhua, C., et al. (2012). Reproductive variables and risk of breast malignant and benign tumours in Yunnan Province, China. *Asian Pacific Journal of Cancer Prevention, 13,* 2179–2184.

Yokoyama, Y., Ueda, T., Irahara, M., & Aono, T. (1994). Releases of oxytocin and prolactin during breast massage and suckling in puerperal women. *European Journal of Obstetrics, Gynecology and Reproductive Biology, 53,* 17–20.

Zanin, E., et al. (2011). White matter maturation of normal human fetal brain. An in vivo diffusion tensor tractography study. *Brain Behavior, 1,* 95–108. doi: 10.1002/brb3.17

Zhao, J., Gonzalez, F., & Mu, D. (2011). Apnea of prematurity: From cause to treatment. *European Journal of Pediatrics, 170,* 1097–1105. doi: 10.1007/s00431-011-1409-6

Ziegler, A.G., et al. (2012). Long-term protective effect of lactation on the development of type 2 diabetes in women with recent gestational diabetes mellitus. *Diabetes, 61,* 3167–3171. doi: 10.2337/db12-0393

Zuppa, A.A., Tornesello, A., Papacci, P., Tortorolo, G., Segni, G., Lafuenti, G., … & Carta, S. (1988). Relationship between maternal parity, basal prolactin levels and neonatal breast milk intake. *Biology of the Neonate, 53,* 144–147.

Additional Reading

Academy of Breastfeeding Medicine. (2006). *Clinical protocol #1: Guidelines for glucose monitoring and treatment of hypoglycemia in breastfed neonates.* Accessed online at http://www.bfmed.org

Academy of Breastfeeding Medicine. (2007). *Clinical protocol #2: Guidelines for hospital discharge of the breastfeeding term newborn and mother: "The Going Home Protocol."* Accessed online at http://www.bfmed.org

Academy of Breastfeeding Medicine. (2009). *Clinical protocol #3: Hospital guidelines for the use of supplementary feedings in the healthy term breastfed neonate.* Accessed online at http://www.bfmed.org

Academy of Breastfeeding Medicine. (2010) *Clinical protocol #7: Model breastfeeding policy.* Accessed online at http://www.bfmed.org

Academy of Breastfeeding Medicine. (2010). *Clinical protocol #22: Guidelines for management of jaundice in the breastfeeding infant equal to or greater than 35 weeks gestation.* Accessed online at http://www.bfmed.org

Adams-Chapman, I. (2006). Neurodevelopmental outcome of the late preterm infant. *Clinics in Perinatology, 33,* 947–964.

Ali, R., Ahmed, S., Qadir, M., & Ahmed, K. (2012). Icterus neonatorum in near-term and term infants. *Sultan Qabos University Medical Journal, 12,* 153–160.

Allen, J., & Hector, D. (2005). Benefits of breastfeeding. *New South Wales Public Health Bulletin, 16,* 42–46.

American Academy of Pediatrics, Committee on Fetus and Newborn. (2011). Postnatal glucose homeostasis in late-preterm and term infants. *Pediatrics, 127,* 575–579. doi: 10.1542/peds.2010-3851

American Academy of Pediatrics, Section on Breastfeeding. (2012). Policy statement: Breastfeeding and the use of human milk. *Pediatrics, 129,* e827–e841. doi: 10.1542/peds.2011-3552

Anadkat, J.S., Kuzniewicz, M.W., Chaudhari, B.P., Cole, F.S., & Hamvas, A. (2012). Increased risk for respiratory distress among white, male, late preterm and term infants. *Journal of Perinatology, 32,* 780–785. doi: 10.1038/jp.2011.191

Anand, K., J.S. & Hickey, P.R. (1987). Pain and its effects in the human neonate and fetus. *New England Journal of Medicine, 317,* 1321–1329.

Araújo, B.F., et al. (2012). Analysis of neonatal morbidity and mortality in late-preterm newborn infants. *Journal of Pediatrics, 88,* 259-266. doi: 10.2223/JPED.2196

Asakura, H. (2004). Fetal and neonatal thermoregulation. *Journal of Nippon Medical School, 71,* 360–370.

Baruah, M.P., Ammini, A.C., & Khurana, M.L. (2001). Demographic, breast-feeding, and nutritional trends among children with type 1 diabetes mellitus. *Indian Journal of Endocrinology and Metabolism, 15,* 38–42. doi: 10.4103/2230-8210.77583

Battineni, S., & Clarke, P. (2012). Green teeth are a late complication of prolonged conjugated hyperbilirubinemia in extremely low birthweight infants. *Journal of Pediatric Dentistry, 34,* 103–106.

Berger, I., Weintraub, V., Kopolovitz, R., & Dollberg, S. (2008). Energy expenditure in breastfed and bottle-fed preterm infants. *Archives of Disease in Childhood, 93,* 241.

Biancuzzo, M. (2003) *Breastfeeding the Newborn* (2nd ed.) St Louis, MO: Mosby.

Bu'Lock, F., Woolridge, M.W., & Baum, J.D. (1990). Development of co-ordination of sucking, swallowing and breathing: Ultrasound study of term and preterm infants. *Developmental Medicine and Child Neurology, 32,* 669–678.

Burgos, A.E., Schmitt, S.K., Stevenson, D.K., & Phibbs, C.S. (2008). Readmission for neonatal jaundice in California, 1991-2000: Trends and implications. *Pediatrics, 121,* e864-869. doi: 10.1542/peds.2007-1214

Capuco, A.V., Connor, E.E., & Wood, D.L. (2008). Regulation of mammary gland sensitivity to thyroid hormones during the transition from pregnancy to lactation. *Experimental Biology and Medicine, 233,* 1309–1314. doi: 10.3181/0803-RM-85

Caspi, A., Williams, B., Kim-Cohen, J., Craig, I.W., Milne, B.J., Poulton, R., . . . & Moffitt, T.E. (2008). Moderation of breastfeeding effects on the IQ by genetic variation in fatty acid metabolism. *Archives of General Psychiatry, 65,* 578–584.

Catalano, P.M., & Sacks, D.A. (2011). Timing of indicated late preterm and early-term birth in chronic medical complications: Diabetes. *Seminars in Perinatology, 35,* 297–301. doi: 10.1053/j.semperi.2011.05.003

Celik, I.H., Demirel, G., Canpolat, F.E., & Dilmen, U. (2013). A common problem for neonatal intensive care units: late preterm infants: A prospective study with term controls in a large perinatal center. *Journal of Maternal, Fetal, and Neonatal Medicine, 26,* 459–462. doi: 10.3109/14767058.2012.735994

Chandra, R.K. (1978). Immunological aspects of human milk. *Nutrition Reviews, 36,* 265–272.

Chapman, D.J. (2011). New evidence: Exclusive breastfeeding and reduced sudden infant death syndrome risk. *Journal of Human Lactation, 27,* 404-405. doi: 10.1177/0890334411420059

Chapman, D.J., & Pérez-Escamilla, R.R. (1999). Identification of risk factors for delayed onset of lactation. *Journal of the American Dietetic Association, 99,* 5.

Chen, C.H., Wang, T.M., Chang, H.M., & Chi, C.S. (2000). The effect of breast- and bottle feeding on oxygen saturation and body temperature in preterm infants. *Journal of Human Lactation, 16,* 21–27.

Clark, R.H. (2005). The epidemiology of respiratory failure in neonates born at an estimated gestational age of 34 weeks or more. *Journal of Perinatology, 25,* 251–257.

Cleaveland, K. (2010). Feeding challenges in the late preterm infant. *Neonatal Network, 29,* 37–41.

Cooke, M., Sheehan, A., & Schmied, V. (2003). A description of the relationship between breastfeeding experiences, breastfeeding satisfaction, and weaning in the first 3 months after birth. *Journal of Human Lactation, 19,* 145–156.

Copland, I., & Post, M. (2004). Lung development and fetal lung growth. *Paediatric Respiratory Reviews, 5,* S259–S264.

Crump, C., Winkleby, M.A., Sundquist, K., & Sundquist, J. (2011). Risk of diabetes among young adults born preterm in Sweden. *Diabetes Care, 34,* 1109–1113. doi: 10.2337/dc10-2108

Davidoff, M.J., et al. (2006). Changes in the gestational age distribution among U.S. singleton births: Impact on rates of late preterm births, 1992-2002. *Seminars in Perinatology, 30,* 8-15.

DeCarvalho, M., Robertson, S., Friedman, A., & Klaus, M. (1983). Effect of frequent breast-feeding on early milk production and infant weight gain. *Pediatrics, 72,* 307–311.

Dennis, C.L. (2003). The breastfeeding self-efficacy scale: Psychometric assessment of the short form. *Journal of Obstetric, Gynecologic and Neonatal Nursing, 32,* 734–744.

Dobak,W.J., & Gardner, M.O. (2006). Late preterm gestation: physiology of labor and implications for delivery. *Clinics in Perinatology, 33,* 765–766.

Emde, R.N., Swedberg, J., & Suzuki, B. (1975). Human wakefulness and biological rhythms after birth. *Archives of General Psychiatry, 32,* 780–783.

Escobar, G.J., Clark, R.H., & Greene, J.D. (2006). Short-term outcomes of infants born at 35 and 36 weeks gestation: We need to ask more questions. *Seminars in Perinatology, 30,* 28–33.

Fairfax, J., & Hector, D. (2005). Benefits of breastfeeding. *New South Wales Public Health Bulletin, 16,* 42–46.

Febo, M., Numan, M., & Ferris, C.F. (2005). Functional magnetic resonance imaging shows oxytocin activates brain regions associated with mother-pup bonding during suckling. *The Journal of Neuroscience, 25,* 11637–11644. doi: 10.1523/JNEUROSCI.3604-05.2005

Gamboni, S.E., Allen, K.J., & Nixon, R.L. (2012). Infant feeding and the development of food allergies and atopic eczema: An update. *Australasian Journal of Dermatology.* Epub ahead of print, October 22, 2012. doi: 10.1111/j.1440-0960.2012.00950.x

Garg, M., & Devaskar, S.U. (2006). Glucose metabolism in the late preterm infant. *Clinics in Perinatology, 33,* 853–857.

Gartner, L.M., et al. (2005). Breastfeeding and the use of human milk. *Pediatrics, 115,* 496–506.

Gioiosa, R. (1964). Breast feeding and child spacing. *Child and Family, 3,* 3–11.

Girard, N., Raybaud, C., & Pon, M. (1995). In vivo MR study of brain maturation in normal fetuses. *American Journal of Neuroradiology, 16,* 407–413.

Grassley, J.S. (2010). Adolescent mothers' breastfeeding social support needs. *Journal of Obstetric, Gynecologic, and Neonatal Nursing, 39,* 713–722. doi: 10.1111/ j.1552-6909.2010.01181.x

Greer, F.R., Sicherer, S.H., Wesley Burks, A., & the Committee on Nutrition and Section on Allergy and Immunology (2008). Effects of early nutritional interventions on the development of atopic disease in infants and children: The role of maternal dietary restriction, breastfeeding, timing of introduction of complementary foods, and hydrolyzed formulas. *Pediatrics, 121,* 183–191. doi: 10.1542/peds.2007-3022

Grimes, D.A., & Economy, K.E. (1995). Primary prevention of gynecologic cancers. *American Journal of Obstetrics and Gynecology, 172,* 227–235.

Gubler, T., Krähenmann, F., Roos, M., Zimmermann, R., & Ochsenbein-Kölble, N. (2012) Determinants of successful breastfeeding initiation in healthy term singletons: A Swiss university hospital observational study. *Journal of Perinatal Medicine.* Epub ahead of print, October 25, 2012. doi:10.1515/jpm-2012-0102

Heinig, M.J. (2001). Host defense benefits of breastfeeding for the infant: Effect of breastfeeding duration and exclusivity. *Pediatric Clinics of North America, 4,* 105–123.

Hilson, J.A., Rasmussen, K.M., & Kjolhede, C.L.(2004). High prepregnant body mass index is associated with poor lactation outcomes among white, rural women independent of psychosocial and demographic correlates. *Journal of Human Lactation, 20,* 18–29. doi: 10.1177/0890334403261345

Huang, A., Tai, B.C., Wong, L.Y., Lee, J., & Yong, E.L. (2009). Differential risk for early breastfeeding jaundice in a multi-ethnic Asian cohort. *Annals of the Academy of Medicine, Singapore, 38,* 217–224.

Huang, M.J., et al. (2004). Risk factors for severe hyperbilirubinemia in neonates. *Pediatric Research, 56,* 682–689.

Hurst, N.M. (2007). Recognizing and treating delayed or failed lactaogenesis II. *Journal of Midwifery and Women's Health, 52,* 588–594.

Jaiin, S., & Cheng, J. (2006). Emergency department visits and rehospitalizations in late preterm infants. *Clinics in Perinatology, 33,* 935–945.

Jaiswal, A., Murki, S., Gaddam, P., & Reddy, A. (2011). Early neonatal morbidities in late preterm infants. *Indian Pediatrics, 48,* 607–611.

Jevitt, C., Hernandez, I., & Groër, M. (2007). Lactation complicated by overweight and obesity: Supporting the mother and newborn. *Journal of Midwifery and Women's Health, 52,* 606–613.

Jorgensen, A.M. (2008). Late preterm birth: a rising trend: part one of a two-part series. *Nursing for Women's Health, 12,* 308–315. doi: 10.1111/j.1751-486X. 2008.00352.x

Karl, D.J. (2004). Using principles of newborn behavioral state of organization to facilitate breastfeeding. *The American Journal of Maternal Child Nursing, 29,* 292–298.

Kent, J.C., Mitoulas, L.R., Cregan, M.D., Geddes, D.T., Larsson, M., Doherty, D.A., & Hartmann, P.E. (2008). Importance of vacuum for breastmilk expression. *Breastfeeding Medicine, 3,* 11–19. doi: 10.1089/bfm.2007.0028

Keren, R., Tremont, K., Luan, X., & Cnaan, A. (2009). Visual assessment of jaundice in term and late preterm infants. *Archives of Disease in Children. Fetal and Neonatal Edition, 94,* F317–F322. doi: 10.1136/adc.2008.150714

Kersula, D.M. (2008). *Breastfeeding: New strategies for improved outcomes.* Eau Claire, WI: PESI Healthcare.

Khashu, M., Narayanan, M., Bhargava, S., & Osiovich, H. (2009). Perinatal outcomes associated with preterm birth at 33 to 36 weeks' gestation: A population-based cohort study. *Pediatrics, 123,* 109–113. doi: 10.1542/peds.2007-3743

Kinney, H.C. (2006). The near-term (late preterm) human brain and risk for periventricular leukomalacia: A review. *Seminars in Perinatology, 30,* 81–88.

Laptook, A., & Jackson, G.l. (2006). Cold stress and hypoglycemia in the late preterm ("near-term") infant: Impact on nursery of admission. *Seminars in Perinatology, 30,* 24–27.

Leonard, L.G. (2002). Breastfeeding higher order multiples: Enhancing support during the postpartum hospitalization period. *Journal of Human Lactation, 18,* 386–392. doi: 10.1177/089033402237914

Li, R., Fein, S.B., & Grummer-Strawn, L.M. (2010). Do infants fed from bottles lack self-regulation of milk intake compared with directly breastfed infants? *Pediatrics, 125,* e1386–e1393. doi: 10.1542/peds.2009-2549

Long, J., Zhang, S., Fang, X., Luo, Y, & Liu, J. (2011). Neonatal hyperbilirubinemia and gly71arg mutation of ugt1a1 gene: A Chinese case-control study followed by systematic review of existing evidence. *Acta Paediatrica,* 100, 966–971. doi: 10.1111/j.1651-2227.2011.02176.x

Lumley, J. (2003). Defining the problem: The epidemiology of preterm birth. *BJOG-an International Journal of Obstetrics and Gynaecology,* 110, 3–7.

Maisels, M.J. (2006). What's in a name? physiologic and pathologic jaundice: The conundrum of defining normal bilirubin levels in the newborn. *Pediatrics, 118,* 805–807. doi: 10.1542/peds.2006-0675

Mannel, R., Martens, P.J., & Walker, M. (2008). *Core Curriculum for Lactation Consultant Practice. International Lactation Consultant Association* (2nd ed.) Sudbury, MA: Jones and Bartlett.

Martin., R.M., et al. (2013). Effects of promoting longer-term and exclusive breastfeeding on adiposity and insulin-like growth factor-l at 11.5 years: A randomized trial. *Journal of the American Medical Association, 309,* 1005–1013. doi: 10.1001/jama.2013.167

McBain, D. (2010). Medical minutes: Breastfeeding baby is healthiest option for new moms. Accessed at http://www.pressandguide.com/articles/2010/09/03/life/doc4c812edc36a4a446333565.txt

McDonald, S.W., Benzies, K.M., Gallant, J.E., McNeil, D.A., Dolan, S.M., & Tough, S.C. (2012). A comparison between late preterm and term infants on breastfeeding and maternal mental health. *Maternal Child Health Journal.* Epub ahead of print, October 7, 2012. doi: 10.1007/s10995-012-1153-1

McLaurin, K.K., Hall, C.B., Jackson, E.A., Owens, O.V., & Mahadevia, P.J. (2009). Persistence of morbidity and cost differences between late-preterm and term infants during the first year of life. *Pediatrics, 123,* 653-659. doi: 10.1542/peds.2008-1439

Meier, P. (1988). Bottle- and breast-feeding: Effects on transcutaneous oxygen pressure and temperature in preterm infants. *Nursing Research, 37,* 36-41.

Mennella, J.A., & Pepino, M.Y. (2010). Breastfeeding and prolactin levels in lactating women with a family history of alcoholism. *Pediatrics, 125,* e1162–e1170. doi: 10.1542/peds.2009-3040

Munakata, S. (2013). Gray matter volumetric MRI differences late-preterm and term infants. *Brain and Development, 35,* 10–16. doi: 10.1016/j.braindev.2011.12.011

Newcomb, P.A., & Trentham-Dietz, A. (2000). Breast feeding practices in relation to endometrial cancer risk, USA. *Cancer Causes and Control, 11,* 663–667.

Newman, J. (2009). *Finger feeding and cup feeding.* Accessed at http://www.breastfeedingonline.com/newman.shtml

O'Connor, M. (1998). *Breastfeeding basics: Growth and development.* Online course available at http://www.breastfeedingbasics.org

Okamura, C., Tsubono, Y., Ito, K., Niikura, H., Takano, T., Nagase, S., Yoshinaga, K., . . . & Yaegashi, N. (2006). Lactation and risk of endometrial cancer in Japan: A case-control study. *Tohoku Journal of Experimental Medicine, 208,* 109–115.

Perrine, C.G., Scanlon, K.S., Li, R., Odom, E., & Grummer-Strawn, L.M. (2012). Baby-friendly hospital practices and meeting exclusive breastfeeding intention. *Pediatrics, 130,* 54–60. doi: 10.1542/peds.2011-3633

Pitcher, J.B., et al. (2012). Physiological evidence consistent with reduced neuro-plasticity in human adolescents born preterm. *Journal of Neuroscience, 32,* 16410–16416. doi: 10.1523/jneurosci.3079-12.2012

Power, M.L., Henderson, Z., Behler, J.E., & Schulkin, J. (2013). Attitudes and practices regarding late preterm birth among American obstetrician-gynecologists. *Journal of Women's Health, 22,* 167–172. doi: 10.1089/jwh.2012.3814

Rich-Edwards, J.W., et al. (2004). Breastfeeding during infancy and the risk of cardiovascular disease in adulthood. *Journal of Epidemiology, 15,* 550–556.

Riman, T., et al. (2002). Risk factors for invasive epithelial ovarian cancer: Results from a Swedish case-control study. *American Journal of Epidemiology, 156,* 363–373.

Rogers, C.E., Lenze, S.N., & Luby, J.L. (2013). Late preterm birth, maternal depression, and risk of preschool psychiatric disorders. *Journal of the American Academy of Child and Adolescent Psychiatry, 52,* 309–318. doi: 10.1016/j.jaac.2012.12.005

Rosenblatt, K.A., & Thomas, D.B. (1995). Prolonged lactation and endometrial cancer. W.H.O. collaborative study of neoplasia and steroid contraceptives. *International Journal of Epidemiology, 24,* 499–503.

Ruth, C.A., Roos, N., Hildes-Ripstein, E., & Brownell, M. (2012). The influence of gestational age and socioeconomic status on neonatal outcomes in late preterm and early term gestation: A population based study. *Biomed Central Pregnancy & Childbirth, 12,* 62. doi: 10.1186/1471-2393-12-62

Salone, L.R., Vann, W.F., & Dee, D.L. (2013). Breastfeeding: An overview of oral and general health benefits. *The Journal of the American Dental Association, 144,* 143–151.

Schubiger, G., Schwartz, U., & Tönz, O. (1997). UNICEF/WHO baby-friendly hospital initiative: Does the use of bottles and pacifiers in the neonatal nursery prevent successful breastfeeding? *European Journal of Pediatrics, 156,* 874–877.

Schwartz, H.P., Haberman, B.E., & Ruddy, R.M. (2011). Hyperbilirubinemia: Current guidelines and emerging therapies. *Pediatric Emergency Care, 27,* 884–889. doi: 10.1097/PEC.0b013e31822c9b4c

Sealy, C.N. (1996). Rethinking the use of nipple shields. *Journal of Human Lactation, 12,* 299–300.

Shiva, M. (1991). Of human rights and women's health. *Women's Global Network for Reproductive Rights, 36,* 55–-57.

Singh, R., et al. (2012). Breastfeeding as a time-varying-time-dependent factor for birth spacing: Multivariate models with validations and predictions. *World Health & Population, 13,* 28-51.

Sloan, S., Stewart, M.C., & Dunne, L.M. (2008). Breastfeeding promotes infant cognitive development, independent of socioeconomic factors and stimulation in the home. *Archives of Disease in Childhood, 93,* 32.

Spatz, D.L. (2011). Innovations in the provision of human milk and breastfeeding for infants requiring intensive care. *Journal of Obstetric, Gynecologic, and Neonatal Nursing,* 1-6. doi: 10.1111/j.1552-6909.2011.01315.x

Speller, E., Brodribb, W., & McGuire, E. (2012). Breastfeeding and thyroid disease: A literature review. *Breastfeeding Review, 20,* 41–47.

Stevenson, D.K., Dennery, P.A., & Hintz, S.R. (2001). Understanding newborn jaundice. *Journal of Perinatology, 21,* S21–S24.

Strode, M.A., Dewey, K.G., & Lönnerdal, B. (1986). Effects of short-term caloric restriction on lactational performance of well-nourished women. *Acta Paediatrica Scandinavica, 75,* 222–229.

Stuebe, A. (2009). The risks of not breastfeeding for mothers and infants. *Reviews in Obstetrics and Gynecology, 2 ,*222-231.

Stuebe, A.M., Willet, W.C., Xue, F., & Michels, K.B. (1995). Lactation and incidence of premenopausal breast cancer: A longitudinal study. *Archives of Internal Medicine, 169,* 1364–1371. doi: 10.1001/archinternmed.2009.231

Sweet, L. (2008). Expressed breast milk as "connection" and its influence on the construction of "motherhood" for mothers of preterm infants: A qualitative study. *International Breastfeeding Journal, 3,* 30. doi: 10.1186/1746-4358-3-30

Talge, N.M. (2012). Late-preterm birth by delivery circumstances and its association with parent-reported attention problems in childhood. *Journal of Developmental and Behavioral Pediatrics, 33,* 405–415. doi: 10.1097/DBP.0b013e3182564704

Tanaka, S., Mito, T., & Takashima, S. (1995). Progress of myelination in the human fetal spinal nerve roots, spinal cord and brainstem with myelin basic protein immunohistochemistry. *Early Human Development, 41,* 49–59.

Tomashek, K.M., Shapiro-Mendoza, C.K., Davidoff, M.J., & Petrini, J.R. (2007). Differences in mortality between late-preterm and term singleton infants in the United States, 1995–2002. (2007). *Journal of Pediatrics, 151,* 450–456.

Tozzi, A.E., et al. (2012). Effect of duration of breastfeeding on neuropsychological development at 10 to 12 years of age in a cohort of healthy children. *Developmental Medicine and Child Neurology, 54,* 843–848. Doi: 10.1111/j.1469-8749.2012.04319.x

Trout, K.K., Averbuch, T., & Barowski, M. (2011). Promoting breastfeeding among obese women and women with gestational diabetes mellitus. *Current Diabetes Report, 11,* 7–12. doi: 10.1007/s11892-010-0159-6

Tung, K, et al. (2003). Reproductive factors and epithelial ovarian cancer risk by histologic type: A multiethnic case-control study. *American Journal of Epidemiology, 158 ,* 629–638.

Veena, S.R., et al. (2010). Infant feeding practice and childhood cognitive performance in South India. *Archives of Disease in Childhood, 95,* 347–354. doi: 10.1136/adc.2009.165159

Ward Platt, M., & Deshpande, S. (2005). Metabolic adaptation at birth. *Seminars in Fetal and Neonatal Medicine, 10,* 341–350.

Wasser, D.E., & Hershkovitz, I. (2010). The question of ethnic variability and the Darwinian significance of physiological neonatal jaundice in East Asian populations. *Medical Hypotheses, 75,* 187–189. doi:10.1016/j.mehy.2010.02.017

Watchko, J.F., et al. (2009). Complex multifactorial nature of significant hyperbilirubinemia in neonates. *Pediatrics, 124,* e868–877. doi: 10.1542/peds.2009-0460

Wight, N.E. (2003). Breastfeeding the borderline (near-term) preterm infant. *Pediatric Annals, 32,* 329–336.

Wojcicki, J.M. (2011). Maternal prepregnancy body mass index and initiation and duration of breastfeeding: A review of the literature. *Journal of Women's Health, 20,* 341–347. doi: 10.1089/wh.2010.2248

Yazawa, M., Watanabe, M., So, M., & Kishi, K. (2013). Treatment of congenital absence of the mammary gland. *Case Reports in Surgery,* doi: 10.1155/2013/676573

Zinaman, M.J., Hughes, V., Queenan, J.T., Labbok, M.H., & Albertson, B. (1992). Acute prolactin and oxytocin responses and milk yield to infant suckling and artificial methods of expression in lactating women. *Pediatrics, 89,* 437–440.

Zuppa, A.A., Catenazzi, P., Orchi, C., Cota, F., Calabrese, V., Cavani, M., & Romagnoli, C. (2013). Hyperbilirubinemia in healthy newborns born to immigrant mothers from southeastern Asia compared to Italian ones. *Indian Journal of Pediatrics.* Epub ahead of print, January 10, 2013.

Resources for Nurses and Parents

Academy of Breastfeeding Medicine

- Worldwide organization of physicians dedicated to the promotion, protection, and support of breastfeeding and human lactation
www.bfmed.org
- Academy of Breastfeeding Medicine protocol #10: Breastfeeding the late preterm infant (34 0/7 to 36 6/7 Weeks Gestation)
www.bfmed.org/Media/Files/Protocols?Protocol%2010%20 Revised%20English%206.11.pdf

Ameda

- Downloadable tools for clinicians
www.ameda.com/ameda-support-tools/clinical-tools

American Academy of Pediatrics

- Breastfeeding initiatives and information for clinicians, including policies, resources for office and hospital, and current research
2.aap.org/breastfeeding/healthProfessionalsResourceGuide.html

AWHONN: Association of Women's Health, Obstetric, and Neonatal Nurses

- Late Preterm Initiative and information for clinicians and parents
www.awhonn.org/awhonn/contentdo?name=03_Journals PubResearch/3G6_LatePreterm.htm

Baby-Friendly USA

- The accrediting body for the Baby-Friendly Hospital Initiative in the United States
www.babyfriendlyusa.org

Breastfeeding.com

■ All about baby care and feeding, but not specific to late preterm infants
www.breastfeeding.com

Coalition for Improving Maternity Services

■ www.motherfriendly.org

Donor Human Milk Bank

■ Information about receiving or donating breast milk
www.hmbana.org

International Board of Lactation Consultant Examiners

■ Information on becoming an international board-certified lactation consultant (IBCLC)
www.iblce.org/certification

International Childbirth Education Association
www.icea.org

International Lactation Consultant Association

■ Online database of local lactation consultants
www.ilca.org

LactMed

■ A free online database with information on drugs and lactation
www.toxnet.nlm.nih.gov/cgi-bin/sis/htmlgen?LACT

La Leche League International

■ International nonprofit, nonsectarian organization dedicated to providing education, information, support, and encouragement to women who want to breastfeed
www.llli.org

March of Dimes

■ Organization for stronger, healthier babies, especially premature babies
www.marchofdimes.com

Medela

■ Information on insurance reimbursement
www.medelabreastfeedingus.com/breastfeeding-insurance

- Patient teaching handouts for a variety of breastfeeding issues
  www.medelabreastfeedingus.com/for-professionals/lactation-professional-information/literature-and-brochures
- Latest research and technology
  www.medelabreastfeedingus.com/for-professionals/lactation-professional-information/research-and-news-
- Simple explanations for parents
  www.medelabreastfeedingus.com/for-professionals/tips-and-solutions

National Alliance for Breastfeeding Advocacy

- Dedicated to the protection, promotion, and support of breastfeeding in the United States
  www.naba-breastfeeding.org

National Healthy Mothers, Healthy Babies Coalition
www.hmhb.org

National Institute of Health

- United States department for health research
  www.nih.gov

National Organization of Mothers of Twins Clubs
www.nomotc.org

National WIC Association

- Food and nutrition services for low-income women, infants, and children up to age 5
  www.nwica.org

PESI Healthcare

- Continuing education for nurses
  www.pesihealthcare.com

Stanford School of Medicine

- Video of Jane Morton's hand expression technique
  http://newborns.stanford.edu/Breastfeeding?HandExpression.html

United States Breastfeeding Committee

- List of breastfeeding coalitions by state
  www.usbreastfeeding.org

U.S. Department of Health

■ Provides breastfeeding information and other essential human services
www.womenshealth.gov/breastfeeding

U.S. Food and Drug Administration

■ Regulates medical devices such as breast pumps
www.fda.gov/medicaldevices

U.S. Lactation Consultant Association

■ A professional association for IBCLCs and other health care professionals who care for breastfeeding families
www.uslca.org

Wellstart International

■ Nonprofit organization based in San Diego, California, funded by charitable donations and dedicated to optimal mother and infant nutrition worldwide
www.wellstart.org

World Health Organization

■ United Nations public health department
www.who.int/en

YouTube

■ Ameda Purely Yours Breast Pump Custom Fit Flange System video demonstrating correct flange fit
www.youtube.com/watch?v=V1ID5VP65e0
■ *How To Put on Nipple Shields* video, correct nipple shield application technique
youtube.com/watch?v=gIUgmdF6jJM

Index

abnormal fetal heart rate, 11
abruption, 58
Academy of Breastfeeding Medicine
     Protocol 10, 90–91, 148, 163
  inpatient breastfeeding, 91
acidosis, 34
acute bilirubin encephalopathy, 33, 38
ADHD. *See* attention-deficit/
     hyperactivity disorder
adult thermoregulation, 26
advanced maternal age, risks of, 14
  caesarean delivery, 14
  macrosomia, 14
  stillborn births, 14
AGA. *See* appropriate-for-
     gestational-age infant
age, effect on pregnancy, 4
Agency for Healthcare Research and
     Quality, 73
albumin-binding, 37
  sites, 28
albumin-bound bilirubin, 38
  asphyxia, 38
  hyperosmolality, 38
  hypoperfusion, 38
  hypoxia, 38
  sepsis, 38
alcohol, 63
alpha-agonists, 12
alpha-lactalbumin, 74
altered estrogen, 57
altered sleep states, 45
alternate breast feeding, 177
alveolar air spaces, 43

alveolar collapse, 42
alveolarization, 43
alveoli, 43
Ameda nipple shields, 126
American Academy of Pediatrics,
     163
amniotic banding, 11
amniotic fluid volume, 11
anemia, 60
ankyloglossia, 178–179
anterior pituitary ischemia, 58
apnea of prematurity, 44–45
  altered sleep states, 45
  bradycardia, 44–45
  central nervous system
     abnormalities, 45
  contributing factors, 45
     glucose and electrolyte
        imbalances, 45
     hypercapnia, 45
     hyperthermia, 45
     hypoxia, 45
     infections, 45
     magnesium sulfate
        administration, 45
  oxygen desaturation, 44
apnea, 29, 38, 42, 44,
  causes
     carbon dioxide central
        chemosensitivity, 44
     decreased upper airway dilator
        muscle tone, 44
     hypoxic respiratory
        depression, 44

immature pulmonary irritant
  receptors, 44
  laryngeal distortion, 44
appropriate-for-gestational-age
  (AGA) infant, 178
  fatality rate, 177
ART. *See* assisted reproductive
  technology
asphyxia, 38
assisted reproductive technology
  (ART), 14
Association of Women's Health,
  Obstetric and Neonatal
  Nurses, 83
asthma, 12–13, 73
atopic dermatitis, 73
attention-deficit/hyperactivity
  disorder (ADHD), 15
autoimmune disorders, 13
  systemic lupus erythematosus, 13
  thyroid disease, 13
Avent nipple shields, 126

baby–mother separation, 45–46
Baby-Friendly Hospital Initiative,
  81–83, 84, 86
  breast milk alternatives, 85
  International Code of Marketing of
    Breast Milk Substitutes, 81
  Joint Commission's Perinatal
    Care Core Measure Set
    #PC-05, 85
  optimal breastfeeding techniques,
    85–86
  Ten Steps to Successful
    Breastfeeding, 81, 82
bacterial infections, 49
bariatric surgery, 60
  lactogenesis II, 60
  malabsorptive, 60
  restrictive, 60
Beck Depression Inventory, 67
beta-blockers, 12
beta-carotene, 90

bilirubin, 28, 33, 89
  albumin-binding, 37
  breastfeeding, 37–39
  bruising, 33
  clearance, delayed, 162
  conjugation, 35
  delayed peak, 37
  early symptoms, 38
    high-pitched cry, 38
    hypotonia, 38
    lethargy, 38
    poor feeding, 38
  enterohepatic circulation, 37
  G6PD deficiency, 33
  impaired hemolytic processes, 33
  jaundice, 33–36
  kernicterus, 33, 37–38
  late symptoms, 38
  meconium, 37, 38
  polycythemia, 33
  reduction of, 162, 163
  temperature instability, 37
  total serum, 37
  unconjugated levels, 37
  uridine diphosphate glucuronyl
    transferase, 33
birth process, maternal self-esteem
  and, 66–67
birth weights, 13
BMI. *See* body mass index
body mass index (BMI), 14–15, 65, 66
Bottle feeding, 111, 164–166
  advantages, 165
  disadvantages, 165–166
    contamination, 165
    decreased oxygen saturation, 165
    formula temperature, 165
    frequency, 165
    heart rate increases, 165
    maternal self-worth, 165
    physiological stability, 165
    respiratory rate increase, 165
    skin-to-skin contact, 165
  flow of, 165
  infant position while feeding, 165

nipple confusion, 164–165
paced feeding techniques, 165
slow-flow nipples, 165
bradycardia, 42, 44–45
brain dysmaturity, 18
electroencephalographic studies, 18
brain growth, 17
brain dysmaturity, 18
maturation process, 17–19
brain maturation process, 17–19
brain tissue development, 18–19
brainstem development, 18
breastfeeding, 18
cerebellum, 19
cerebral cortex, 19
childhood neuropsychiatric
disorders, 19
external stimulation stress, 22
extra-uterine life, 20
gyri, 22
immature, 20–21
longer gestation, 17–18
magnetic resonance diffusion tensor
imaging, tractography, 19
MRI scans, 17–18
sleep patterns, 18
sulci, 22
synaptogenesis, 19
white matter, 19
brain tissue, development of, 18–19
full term vs. late term baby, 19
myelinated white matter, 19
brainstem development, 18
breast augmentation, 55–56
polyacrylamide hydrogel, 55
silicone implants, 55–56
breast cancer, prevention of, 73–74
alpha-lactalbumin, 74
endometrial cancer, 74
breast compressions, 21, 87, 188
C-hold, 117
colostrum, 21, 115
effective methods, 117–118
hyperbilirubinemia, 115
intraoral vacuum pressure, 115–116

milk removal study, 116–117
milk transfer, 116
positive effects of, 118–119
wake cycles, 115
breast feeding, flange positioning, 149
breast hypoplasia, 54
breast infection
galoctoceles, 55
intraprosthetic collection, 55
breast lift, 56–57
Breast massage, 156
breast milk, 21
alternatives to, 85
flow, 125
jaundice, 35–36
bilirubin conjugation, 35
lipase activity, 35
mechanisms, 35–36
metabolite, 35
normalization of, 36
removal, 169
sodium levels, 60
breast pumping
discontinuing, 144, 151
emptying breasts, 150
breast pumps
basic principles, 137–138
cesarean delivery and, 143
choosing, 148–149
double electric pump, 149
education in, 144, 145
Food and Drug Administration,
descriptions, 138–139
labels, multiple users, 138
Limerick Inc., 139
manual, 149
manufacturer labels, 138–139
hospital grade, 138–139
multiple users, 138
single user, 138
manufacturer research, 139–142
Ameda Inc., 140–141
Elite, test of, 140–141
Hygeia Inc., 142
Limerick Inc., 141

Medela, 139–140
   modified pumping pattern, 140
massage, 143
Medela, 138–139
nipple pain, 145
nipple size, 146
overweight women, 143
prolactin receptors, 143
pumping style, 142–143
regulation of, 138
renting of, 138
research of, 144–145
session length, 150–151
setup and use, 145
   double electric breast
      pump, 145
   pump flange fit, 145
   vacuum pressure, 145
single electric, 149
standards, 142
stress levels, 143
style and outcome, 142–143
   milk expression, 143
   sequential, 142–143
   simultaneous, 142–143
types, 145–146
breastfeeding, 7, 18, 19, 20–21, 22, 25,
      26, 30, 38–39, 42, 45
alternating of, 177
bilirubin, 37
breast compressions, 21
cognitive development, 70
collaborative care, 184
decreased reflexes, 21–22
difficulties in, 11, 12, 15
duration of, 66
emotional satisfaction,
      182–183
emptying of, 150
formula feeding vs., 71–73
hypotonia, 21
impact of consistent care, 183
mother–baby separation, 45–46
   colostrum, 45
nipple shield, 22

perceived risks of, 75
reasons to, 69–75
risks of not breastfeeding,
      69–75
   cancer, 73–74
   financial cost, 73
   hyperbilirubinemia, 71
   impaired neurological
      functioning, 69–70
   infection, 70–71
   jaundice, 71
   metabolic demands, 71
   risk ratios, 73
sharing of, 176
stimulation levels, 22
summaries of, 186–189
   breast compressions, 188
   colostrum, 189
   double electric multiuser pump,
      188
   hand expression, 188
   nipple shields, 188
   parental assistance, 189
   pediatrician follow-up, 189
   proper latch, 187–188
   summaries of, proper
      positioning, 187
   skin-to-skin contact, 187
   supplements, 189
breast reduction, 56–57
breast stimulation, decreased, 162
breastfeeding intervention, 89
   Academy of Breastfeeding
      Medicine, 90–91
   assistance in, 92
   colostrum, 90
   feeding frequency, 89
   feeding volumes, 91
   initiation after birth, 91
   instructions re, 91–92
   outcomes, 89
   weight loss, 89
breastfeeding jaundice, 34–35
breastfeeding patterns, surgical
      effect on, 56

Breastfeeding Self-Efficacy Scale, 66
breastfeeding termination, nipple
    shield effect on, 124
breastfeeding tools
  nipple shields, 181–182
  satisfaction rate, 181–182
breasts, surgery of, 54–55
  augmentation, 55–56
  breast lift, 56–57
  reduction, 56–57
  underdeveloped, 54
breathing issues, nipple shields and,
    127–128
British Columbia Perinatal Database
    Registry, 50
brown fat, 26, 30
  breastfeeding, 30
  efferent nerves, 26
  glucose homeostasis, 30
  glycerol, 30
  hypothalamus, 26
  noradrenalin, 2 6
bruising, 33
buccal fat pads, 124
  lack of, 124, 125
burping, 44

calcium channel blockers, 12
cancer, prevention of, 73–74
  ovarian, 74
carbon dioxide central
    chemosensitivity, 44
cardiac disease, 13
CDC. *See* Centers for Disease Control
    and Prevention
Centers for Disease Control
    and Prevention (CDC),
    14, 73
central nervous system
  abnormalities to, 45
  damage to, 186
cerebellum, growth of, 19
  cortical surface, 19
  neuronal proliferation, 19

cerebral cortex, 19
  dendritic development, 19
  gyral development, 19
  synapsed afferent axonal
    terminals, 19
  volume increase, 19
cesarean delivery, 11, 14, 29, 43, 62
  fetal distress, 43
  hypoglycemia, 62
  milk transfer, 143
  patient-controlled analgesia, 62
  pethidine patient-controlled
    epidural analgesia, 62
  preeclampsia, 43
  respiratory distress, 43
childhood neuropsychiatric
    disorders, 19
childhood obesity, 73
chin stimulus, 109
choking, prevention of, 125
C-hold, 117
cholesterol, 71
chorioamnionitis, 50
chronic fetal hyperinsulinemia, 12
chronic hypertension, 12
chronic intrauterine tissue
    hypoxia, 12
  breastfeeding difficulties, 12
circulating monocytes, 49
clutch position, 112
cognitive development, 70
cognitive development, Philippines
    Nonverbal Intelligence
    Test, 70
collaborative care, 184
colostrum, 21, 45, 63, 70, 87,
    90, 91, 92, 115, 117, 118,
    150,151,155,158, 167, 178
  beta carotene, 90
  energy value, 90
  feeding, 38, 189
  function of, 90
    fibronectin, 90
    interferon, 90
    interleukin-10, 90

lactoferrin, 90
lysozyme epidermal growth
factor, 90
secretory immunoglobulin A, 90
white blood cells, 90
hand expression of, 153, 154
laxative, 90
production, 67
compression pump, 146
conduct disorders, 15
congenital malformations, 11
conjugated bilirubin, 34
consistent care, 183
contact nipple shields, 127–128
breathing issues, 127, 128
Medela, 127–128
contamination, bottles and, 165
cortical surface area, 19
cradle hold, 107
cross-contamination, breast pumps
and, 138
cross-cradle hold, 107–108
crying, 29
cup feeding, 166–167
neonatal intensive care
unit, 167
paladai, 167
cyanosis, 29

"dancer hand" position, 111
dangling limbs, 104
death, risk of, 75
decreased reflexes, 21–22
rooting reflexes, 21
decreasing stimuli, 95
kangaroo care, 95–96
dehydration, 31, 163
dendritic development, 19
diabetes mellitus, 73
diabetes, 12, 28, 29, 59
chronic fetal hyperinsulinemia, 12
chronic intrauterine tissue
hypoxia, 12
hypoglycemia, 12

lactogenesis II, 59
severe neonatal respiratory
failure, 12
direct bilirubin, 34
diuretics, 12
double electric breast pump,
145–146, 149, 154
flange, 145
multiuser, 188
Dr. Brown's nipple shields, 127
dropper, 166

Early Human Development, 115
early term infants, 3
early-onset exaggerated physiologic
jaundice, 37
early-onset sepsis, 50
causes, 51
gram-negative organisms, 51
gram-positive organisms, 51
yeast, 51
risk factors, 51
Hispanic ethnicity, 51
ECG studies. *See*
electroencephalographic
studies
eclampsia, 10
efferent nerves, 26
electroencephalographic (ECG)
studies, 18
electrolyte imbalances, 45
Elite pump, test of, 140–141
emotional care, 182
EnDeare pump, 142
endometrial cancer, 74
energy expenditure, 96, 116
decreasing of, 99–101
limit feeding, 99–100
obnoxious stimuli, 100–101
supplemental feedings, 100
enterohepatic circulation of bilirubin,
37
environmental concerns, risk of
formula feeding, 72–73

epidural analgesia, 61–62
erythroblastosis fetalis, 11
Escherichia coli, 51
evidence-based techniques, 186
expression of colostrum, 87
external stimulation stress, 22
extra-uterine life, adapting to, 20
  breastfeeding, 20
  feeding, 20
  hypotonia, 20
  neurodevelopment maturation, 20
  sleep, 20
eyes, rolling of, 29

fat pads, 124
fatality rates, 177
fat-soluble jaundice, 34
FDA. *See* Food and Drug
    Administration
feeding, 20
  aversion to, 11
  cues, 97–98
  efficiency of, 163
  frequency of, 89
  hypoglycemia's effect on, 29
  limiting of, 99–100
  pillows, 112
  slings, 112
  techniques, paced, 165
  volume of, 91
  supplemental, 100
fetal compression syndrome, 11
fetal distress, 43
fetal heart rate, abnormal, 11
fetal lung fluid, 43
fibronectin, 90
  phagocytes, 90
financial costs, not breastfeeding
    and, 73
  Agency for Healthcare Research
    and Quality, 73
  Centers for Disease Control and
    Prevention, 73
  gastroenteritis, 73

necrotizing enterocolitis, 73
  respiratory tract infections, 73
  SIDS, 73
finger feeding, 168
  syringe, 168
flange, fit, 145, 146
  positioning of, 149
  styles, 147
  hard-rimmed, 147
  soft-rimmed, 147
flow preferences, 165
food and Drug Administration,
    regulations re breast pumps,
    138
football hold, 105–107
formula feeding, risks of,
    71–73
  environment, 72–73
  infants, 71–72
  mothers, 72
formula usage, 162
  protein hydrolysate, 162
formula, temperature of, 165
free fatty acids, 31
French feeding tube, 168
full-term baby
  brain development, 19
  nipple shields, 126
fungal infections, 49

G6PD deficiency, 33
galactoceles, removal of, 55
galactopoietic response, 57
galactosemia, 85
gastroenteritis, 73
gavage feeding, 168
  neonatal intensive care unit, 168
gestation process, effect on brain,
    17–18
  disruptions, 18
  respiratory status, 67–68
gestational diabetes, 12, 28, 29, 57
gluconeogenesis pathway, 28,
    30, 31

glucose, 28, 44, 71, 186
   brain usage, 31
   homeostasis, 30
   imbalances, 45
   levels after birth, 31
   reduction of, 163
   substitutes for, 31
      free fatty acids, 31
      glycerol, 31
      ketone bodies, 31
      lactic acid, 31
   testing, 30
glycerol, 30, 31
   gluconeogenesis pathway, 30
glycogenolysis, 30–31
gram-negative organisms, 51
gram-positive organisms, 51
gryi, 22
gut flora pH level, 162
gyral development, 19

hand expression, 87, 188
   additional milk via, 154–155
   benefits of, 153
   efficiency of, 154
   electric pumps vs., 154
   following birth, 155
   hands-on pumping, 158–159
   influencing milk flow, 156
   techniques, 156–159
      daily practice of, 157
      initiating of, 157
      nipple pain, 157
      Russian, 156, 158
hands-on pumping, 158–159
   *Maximizing Milk Production
      and Hands-On Pumping*,
      158
hard-rimmed flanges, 147
health initiatives
   Baby-Friendly Hospital
      Initiative, 81–83
   definition of, 81
   guidelines, 84, 85

International Code of Marketing
   of Breast-Milk Substitute,
   82–83
late preterm initiatives, 83–84
neonatal intensive care
   unit, 84
heart rate, increase of, 165
HELLP syndrome, 10
hemoglobin, 33, 71
hepatic glycogen, 30
   effect on late preterm infant, 31
higher-order multiples, 175–176
high-pitched cry, 38
hormones, effect on milk supply,
   57–59
   hyperthyroidism, 58
   hypothyroidism, 57–58
   polycystic ovarian syndrome, 57
   retained placental fragments, 58
   Sheehan's syndrome, 58
   theca lutein cysts, 59
hospital-grade breast pumps,
   138–139
hospital readmittance, 6, 7, 50
Hygeia Inc., EnDeare, 142
hyperbilirubinemia, 33, 35, 37,
   38, 39, 71, 85, 115, 163, 185
   early-onset exaggerated
      physiologic jaundice, 37
   occurrences of, 36
   risk factors, 36–37
   suffering by late preterm infants,
      36–37
hypercapnia, 45
hypernatremic dehydration, 60
hyperosmolality, 38
hypertension, 12
   gestational diabetes, 12
hypertension, placental
   abruption, 12
   preeclampsia, 12
   treatments, 12
      alpha-agonists, 12
      beta-blockers, 12
      calcium channel blockers, 12

diuretics, 12
vasodilators, 12
hyperthermia, 25, 38, 44, 45
  breastfeeding, 25
  sepsis, 25
hyperthyroidism
  liver metabolism, 58
  mammary lipid metabolism, 58
  oxytocin, 58
hypoglycemia, 12, 25, 27, 28, 37,
    51, 62, 85, 163, 178, 185
  cesarean section, 29
  factors in, 28
  gestational diabetes, 29
  glucose testing, 30
  late preterm vs. normal
    newborns, 29
  risk factors, 28–29
  symptoms, 29–30
    apnea, 29
    cyanosis, 29
    exaggerated Moro reflex, 29
    eyes rolling, 29
    high-pitched or weak crying, 29
    hypothermia, 29
    hypotonia, 29
    lethargy, 29
    poor feeding, 29
    seizures, 29
    tachypnea, 29
    tremors, 29
hypoperfusion, 38
hypopituitarism, 58
hypoplastic breasts, 54
hypotension, 58
hypothalamus, 26
hypothermia, 25, 27, 29, 34, 37, 45,
    163, 185
  breastfeeding, 27
  gestational diabetes, 28
  hypoglycemia, 27
  lactic acid accumulation, 45
  metabolic acidosis, 45
  risk of, 28
  sepsis, 25

hypothyroidism, 57–58
  serum oxytocin concentrations, 57
  thyroid, 57
hypotonia, 20, 21, 29, 38, 44, 112
hypotonic condition, 27
hypotonic jaw, 111
hypovolemia, 60
hypoxia, 34, 37, 38, 45
hypoxic respiratory depression, 44

immature brain maturation,
    20–21
  breastfeeding, 20–21
immature pulmonary irritant
    receptors, 44
immunity, 49
impaired hemolytic processes, 33
impaired neurological functioning,
    69–70
indirect bilirubin, 34
infants
  brain, lactate metabolization, 31
  position during feeding, 165
  risks from formula feeding,
    71–72
  vulnerability of, 87
infections, 45, 70–71
  bacterial, 49
  British Columbia Perinatal
    Database Registry, 50
  fungal, 49
  hospital readmissions, 50
  incidents of, 49
  jaundice, 50
  Massachusetts General Hospital,
    49–51
infertility treatment, 13–14
  assisted reproductive
    technology, 14
inpatient breastfeeding, 91
insufficient milk supply, 53
insulin resistance, 57
insulin, 71
interferon, 90

interleukin-10, 90
international Code of Marketing of
    Breast Milk Substitutes, 81, 82–83
intraoral vacuum pressure, 115–116,
    124
    Early Human Development, 115
    energy expenditure, importance
        of, 116
    measuring of, 116
    Pascal's law, 116
intrapartum intravenous fluid
    administration, 62–63
intraprothetic collection, sterile
    pus, 55
intrauterine growth retardation
    (IUGR), 11
intrauterine-growth-restricted
    (IUGR) infant, 178
    hypoglycemia, 178
    risks, 178
intraventricular hemorrhage, 178
IUGR. *See* intrauterine-growth-
    restricted infant

jaundice, 11, 28, 33, 34–36, 50, 51,
    71, 161
    albumin-binding sites, 28
    bilirubin, 28
    breast milk, 35–36
    breastfeeding, 34–35
    early-onset exaggerated
        physiologic, 37
    pathological, 34
    physiological, 34
Joint Commission's Perinatal
    Care Core Measure Set
    #PC-05, 85
*Journal of Obstetric, Gynecologic and
    Neonatal Nursing*, 98
Journal of Perinatology, 6
jury duty, 69

kangaroo care, 95–96
    skin-to-skin contact, 95, 96–98

kernicterus (acute bilirubin
    encephalopathy), 33,
    37–38, 39
    albumin, 38
    causes of, 38
        unconjugated bilirubin levels, 38
        unbound lipid-soluble
            bilirubin, 38
ketone bodies, 31

lactate metabolization, 31
lactation, absence of, 58
lactic acid, 27, 31
    accumulation, 45
lactoferrin, 90
lactogenesis II, 37, 58, 59, 60, 61,
    140, 145, 161
    delay of, 162
Lancet, The, 5
lap banding, 60
    lactogenesis II, 60
laryngeal distortion, 44, 46
    causes of, 46
    obstructive apnea, 46
    prevention of, 46
latching, 109–111, 132–134,
    187–188
    actual positioning, 111
    baby's mouth, 132–133
    chin stimulus, 109
    mouth-to-nipple positioning, 110
    nipple shield, 111
    nose-to-nipple technique, 111
    philtrum-to-nipple positioning, 111
    sandwich technique, 110
late preterm infant
    brain development, 19
    breastfeeding, 7
    causes, 9, 10–16
    complications, 6–7
    costs of, 5
    definition of, 3
    hospital readmittance, 6
    morbidity rates, 5–6

nipple shields, 126
nomenclature adoption of, 4
late preterm initiatives, 83–84
　Association of Women's Health,
　　Obstetric and Neonatal
　　Nurses, 83
　National Perinatal Association,
　　83–84
　physician groups, 83
late term deliveries
　incidence of, 4
　decline in, 4
　effect of age, 4
　race, 4
　worldwide statistics, 4, 5
late-onset sepsis, 50
　causes
　　gram-negative organisms, 51
　　gram-positive organisms, 51
　　mother's age, 51
　organisms, 51
　　Escherichia coli, 51
　　Staphylococcus aureus, 51
laxative, 90
lethargy, 29, 38, 51
leukemia, 73
Limerick Inc.
　hospital grade breast pumps, 139
　PJ's Comfort pump, 141–142
Limerick pump, 146, 147, 148
　compression, 146
　vacuum, 146
lipase activity, 35
lipid metabolism, 58
liver metabolism, 58
long-term complications, 6
low birth weight, feeding of, 177–178
low milk supply, overweight
　females, 65–66
lungs, development of, 43
　alveoli, 43
　saccular phase, 43
　transition, 43
lysozyme epidermal growth
　factor, 90

macrosomia, 14
magnesium sulfate
　administration of, 45
　effects of, 10
magnetic resonance diffusion
　tensor imaging
　tractography, 19
malabsorptive weight reduction
　surgery, 60
mammary lipid metabolism, 58
manual breast pumps, 149
massachusetts General Hospital,
　49–51
massage, 143
　breasts, 150
mastitis, 135
maternal medical conditions, 10–16
　advanced maternal age, 14
　asthma, 12–13
　autoimmune disorders, 13
　cardiac disease, 13
　chronic hypertension, 12
　diabetes, 12
　infertility treatment, 13–14
　multiple births, 14
　obesity, 14–15
　oligohydramnios, 11
　placenta abruption, 10–11
　preeclampsia, 10
　previous preterm birth, 16
　renal disease, 13
　Rh disease, 11
　smoking, 15
maternal oxytocin (Pitocin), 34
maternal self-esteem
　factors re, 65, 165
　low milk supply, 65–67
　　Beck Depression Inventory, 67
　　birth process, 66–767
　　breastfeeding duration, 66
　　Breastfeeding Self-Efficacy
　　　Scale, 66
　　colostrum production, 67
　　education re, 67–68
　　gestation, 67

Perception of Insufficient
Milk questionnaire, 65
State-Trait Anxiety
Inventory, 67
Women, Infants, and Children
nutrition program, 66
maternal vitamin B$_{12}$, 60
*Maximizing Milk Production and
Hands-On Pumping*, 158
mechanical pumping, 144
additional milk, 154–155
cessation of, 144
meconium, 37, 71, 89
colostrum feedings, 38
meconium-stained fluid, 11
Medela Inc., 139–140
contact nipple shields, 127–128
hospital grade breast pumps,
138–139
Medela Symphony 2.0 card, 140
nipple shields, 126, 127
pump, 148
Medela Symphony 2.0 card, 140
membrane rupturing, 13
metabolic acidosis, 27, 37, 45
effect on milk supply, 59–60
bariatric surgery, 60
diabetes, 59
lap banding, 60
maternal vitamin B$_{12}$, 60
obesity, 59
postpartum hemorrhage, 60
metabolic demand, 71, 85
cholesterol, 71
glucose, 71
hemoglobin, 71
increase of, 46
insulin, 71
nothing by mouth, 46
transient tachynpea of the
newborn, 46
triglycerides, 71
metabolic disturbances, 34
acidosis, 34
hypothermia, 34

hypoxia, 34
starvation, 34
metabolism, increase of, 31
metabolite, 35
milk expression, 143
sequential, 143
simultaneous pumping, 143
milk flow, 125
hand expression impact on, 156
milk supply
alcohol, 63
breast hypoplasia, 54
breast surgery, 54–55
delay in, 137
establishment of, 137
hormonal
causes, 57–59
issues, 59
insufficient, 53
maternal conditions, 53
maternal self-esteem and, 65–67
medical management issues, 61–63
cesarean section, 62
epidural analgesia, 61–62
intrapartum intravenous fluid
administration, 62–63
lactogenesis II, 61
pitocin induction, 61
metabolic issues, 59–60
nipple
piercing, 54–55
size, 63
short suckling bursts, 53
triplets, 62
twins, 62
weak suck, 53
milk transfer, 116
milk volume, 96
hand expression vs mechanical,
154
modified pumping pattern, 140
Preemie card program, 140
monocytes, 49
sepsis, 49
Staphylococcus epidermidis, 49

morbidity rates, 5–6
Journal of Perinatology, 6
Moro reflex, 29
mother–baby separation, 45–46
mothers
  age, impact on sepsis, 51
  risk of formula feeding, 72
mouth–nipple size mismatch, 179
mouth-to-nipple positioning, 110
MRI scanning, 17–18
Multidisciplinary Guidelines for the
    Care of Late Preterm Infants,
    83–84
multiple births, 14
multiple user breast pump, 138
  cross-contamination, 138
  hospital grade, 138–139
myelin, 19
myelination
  axons, 19
  breastfeeding, 19
  occurrence of, 19
  spinal cord, 19
  synaptic firings, 22
  white matter, 19

National Center for Health Statistics
    (NCHS), 4
National Institute of Child Health
    and Human Development, 3–4
National Perinatal Association, 83–84
  Multidisciplinary Guidelines
    for the Care of Late Preterm
    Infants, 83
NCHS. *See* National Center for
    Health Statistics
near term infants, 3
necrotizing enterocolitis, 73
negative stimuli, reduction of, 97
neonatal intensive care unit (NICU),
    50, 84, 95, 99, 112, 139, 141,
    167, 168,
  discharged from, 85
neonatal morbidity, 42

neonatal respiratory failure, 12
neurodevelopmental maturation, 20
neurological functioning, 69–70
neuronal proliferation, 19
neuropsychiatric disorders, 19
neutral alignment, 104
NICU. *See* neonatal intensive care unit
nipple
  confusion, 164–165, 167
  damage to, 147
  fitting, flange, 146
  flange fit, 145
  height of expansion, 146
  mouth size mismatch, 179
  pain, 145, 146, 157
  piercings, 54–55
  size
    effect on milk supply, 63
    importance of, 146
     height of expansion, 146
  slow-flow, 165
  vacuum pressure, 147–148
nipple shields, 22, 85, 86, 92, 111, 115,
    170, 188
  Avent 126
  Ameda, 126
  controversy over, 121
  satisfaction rate, 181–182
  ultrathin, 121–124
no. 5 French feeding tube, 168
noradrenalin, 26
  oxidation of triglycerides, 26
normal newborns, hypoglycemia
    and, 29
nose-to-nipple technique, 111

obesity, 14–15, 57, 59, 73, 143
  body mass index, 14–15
  breastfeeding difficulties, 15
  preeclampsia, 15
  risks of, 15
obnoxious stimuli, elimination of,
    100–101
obstructive apnea, 46

oligohydramnios, 11
  abnormal fetal heart rate, 11
  amniotic banding, 11
  amniotic fluid volume, 11
  breastfeeding difficulties, 11
  cesarean deliveries, 11
  congenital malformations, 11
  feeding aversion, 11
  fetal compression syndrome, 11
  intrauterine growth retardation, 11
  meconium-stained fluid, 11
  pulmonary hypoplasia, 11
oppositional defiant behavior, 15
optimal breastfeeding techniques,
    85–86
  assistance for, 87
    breast compressions, 87
    colostrum, 87
    expression of colostrum, 87
    hand expression, 87
    pump vacuum, 87
    skin-to-skin contact, 87
    vulnerability, 87
  strategies for, 86–87
    monitoring of, 86–87
optimal positioning, 104–105
otitis media, 73
ovarian cancer, 74
overstimulation, 98–99
  *Journal of Obstetric, Gynecologic and
    Neonatal Nursing*, 98
  signs of, 98–99
  sources of, 99
    neonatal intensive care unit, 99
overweight females, 143
  milk supply and, 65–66
oxygen consumption, 27
  lactic acid, 27
oxygen desaturation, 44
oxygen saturation, 165
oxytocin, 58

PAAG. *See* polyacrylamide hydrogel
  paced feeding techniques, 165

paladai, 167
Pascal's law, 116
pathological jaundice, 34
  conjugated, 34
  direct bilirubin, 34
  risk factors, 34
  unconjugated, 34
  water-soluble bilirubin, 34
patient-controlled analgesia
    (PCA), 62
patient-controlled epidural analgesia
    (PCEA), 62
PCA. *See* patient-controlled
    analgesia
PCEA. *See* patient-controlled
    epidural analgesia
Pediatrix Medical Group, 50
Perception of Insufficient Milk
    questionnaire, 65
periodontal syringes, 166
peristaltic action of the tongue, 124
pethidine (meperidine) patient-
    controlled epidural
    analgesia, 62
pH level of gut flora, 162
phagocytes, 90
Philippines Nonverbal Intelligence
    Test, 70
philtrum-to-nipple positioning, 111
phospholipids, 42
physician group initiatives, 83
physiological jaundice, 34
  fat-soluable, 34
  indirect, 34
  unconjugated, 34
physiological stability, 165
pitocin, 34
pitocin (synthetic oxytocin)
    induction, 61
PJ's Comfort pump, 141–142
placenta abruption, 10–11, 12
  causes, 10
  risk factors, 10–11
  statistics re, 11
placenta expulsion, 58

plunger, 171
pneumonia, 50, 73
polyacrylamide hydrogel (PAAG), 55
polycystic ovarian syndrome
    (PCOS), 57
  altered estrogen, 57
  gestational diabetes, 57
  hypothyroidism, 57
  insulin resistance, 57
  obesity, 57
  preeclampsia, 57
  premature deliveries, 57
polycythemia, 33
polymorphonucleocytes, 90
poor feeding, 38
postpartum hemorrhage, 58, 60
  anemia, 60
  breast milk sodium levels, 60
  hypernatremic dehydration, 60
  hypovolemia, 60
preeclampsia, 10, 12, 13, 15, 43, 57
  eclampsia, 10
  HELLP syndrome, 10
  prophylactic magnesium sulfate, 10
Preemie 1.0 card program, 140
premature deliveries, 57
premature rupture of membranes
    (PROM), 16, 50
preterm births, previous history
    and, 16
prolactin, 57, 58
  levels, 124
  receptors, 143
PROM. *See* premature rupture of
    membranes
Proper feeding positioning
  clutch, 112
  cradle hold, 107
  cross-cradle hold, 107–108
  dancer hand, 111
  dangling limbs, 104
  feeding pillows, 112
  feeding slings, 112
  football hold, 105–107
  methods of, 105–108

  neutral alignment, 104
  optimal, 104–105
  research support of, 103–104
proper positioning
  latch, 109–111
  side-lying positioning, 108
prophylactic magnesium sulfate, 10
protein hydrolysate formula, 162
  bilirubin reduction, 162
  taste of, 162
pulmonary hypoplasia, 11
pulmonary irritant receptors,
    immature, 44
pulmonary vasoconstriction, 27, 45
pump flange fit, 145
pump vacuum, 87

race, effect on pregnancy, 4
reflexes, decreased, 21–22
regular nipple shields, 127–128
  breathing issues, 127–128
  Medela, 127
regulations, breast pumps, 138
renal disease, 13
  birth weights, 13
  preeclampsia, 13
respiratory distress, 51
  apnea of prematurity, 42, 44–45
  bradycardia, 42
  neonatal morbidity, 42
  occurrences of, 41–42
  post-birth, 42
  severe, 45
  surfactant production, 42–43
  transient tachypnea, 42
  types, 43–45
    apnea, 44
    tachypnea, 44
    transient tachypnea, 43
  ventilator-treated respiratory
      distress, 42
respiratory rate, increase of, 165
respiratory status, gestation and, 67–68
respiratory tract infections, 73

restrictive weight reduction
surgery, 60
retained placental fragments, 58
lactogenesis II, 58
prolactin, 58
Rh disease, 11
jaundice, 11
Rh disease. *See also* erythroblastosis
fetalis
risk factors, 10–11, 15, 16, 28–29, 34, 51
hyperbilirbuinemia, 36–37
premature rupture of membranes,
16
supplemental feedings, 166
risk ratios
asthma, 73
atopic dermatitis, 73
childhood obesity, 73
diabetes mellitus, 73
gastroenteritis, 73
leukemia, 73
necrotizing enterocolitis, 73
otitis media, 73
pneumonia, 73
SIDS, 73
rooting reflexes, 21
rupture of membranes, 50
Rush University Medical Center, 139
Russian hand expression techniques,
156, 158

saccular phase, lung development
and, 43
sandwich technique, 110
secretory immunoglobulin A
(sIgA), 90
seizures, 29
self-worth, maternal, 165
sepsis, 25, 38, 44, 45, 49
chorioamnionitis, 50
early-onset, 50
hypoglycemia, 51
hypotonia, 51
jaundice, 51

late-onset, 50
lethargy, 51
neonatal intensive care units, 50
pneumonia, 50
premature rupture of membranes,
50
prevalence of, 50
respiratory distress, 51
Staphylococcus epidermidis, 49
temperature instability, 51
sequential expression, 143
sequential pumping, 142–143
serum oxytocin concentrations, 57
severe respiratory distress, 45
hypothermia, 45
laryngeal distortion, 46
pulmonary vasoconstriction, 45
sepsis, 45
surfactant production, 45
unstable respiratory function, 45
SGA. *See* small-for-gestational-age
infant
Sheehan's syndrome, 58
abruption, 58
absence of lactation, 58
anterior pituitary ischemia, 58
hypopituitarism, 58
hypotension, 58
postpartum hemorrhage, 58
short frenulum, 178–179
short lingual frenulum, 178–179
short suckling bursts, 53
short-term complications, 6
SIDS, 73
sIgA. *See* secretory immunoglobulin
silicone implants, 55–56
simultaneous pumping, 142–143
single electric breast pumps, 149
single electric pumps, 154
single-user breast pump, 138, 139
skin-to-skin contact, 87, 165, 169, 187
benefits of, 96–98
feeding cues, 97–98
milk volume, 96
minimize energy expenditure, 96

negative stimuli reduction, 97
stimuli reduction, 98–99
thermoregulation, 96
mother-infant positions, 97
SLE. *See* systemic lupus
erythematosus
sleep, 20
altered states, 45
patterns, 18
slow-flow nipples, 165
small-for-gestational-age (SGA)
infant, 177–178
fatality rate, 177
smoking, effects of, 15
attention-deficit/hyperactivity
disorder, 15
conduct disorders, 15
oppositional defiant behavior, 15
SNS. *See* Supplemental Nursing
Systems
sodium levels, breast milk and, 60
soft-rimmed flanges, 147
spoon feeding, 167
colostrum, 167
Staphylococcus aureus, 51
Staphylococcus epidermidis, 49
starvation, 34
State-Trait Anxiety Inventory, 67
sterile pus, collection of, 55
stillborn births, 14
stimuli
decreasing of, 95
obnoxious, 100–101
reduction of, 98–99
stress
breast milk and, 143
external stimulation, 22
subcutaneous fat, 26–27
succession feeding, 176
suckling patterns, 125
sulci, 22
supplemental feedings
authorities on, 162–163
Academy of Breastfeeding
Medicine, 163

American Academy of Pediatrics,
163
benefits of, 162–163
delivering of, 161
indications, 163
dehydration, 163
feeding efficiency, 163
hyperbilibubinema, 163
hypoglycemia, 163
hypothermia, 163
weight loss, 163
limiting of, 100
methods, 164–170
bottles, 164–166
cup feeding, 166–167
dropper, 166
finger feeding, 168
gavage, 168
spoon, 167
supplemental nursing systems,
168–172
syringe, 166
protein hydrolysate formula, 162
risks, 166
bilirubin reduction, 163
decreased breast stimulation, 162
decreased glucose, 163
dehydration, 163
delayed bilirubin clearance, 162
formula usage, 162
gut flora pH level, 162
hyperbilirubinemia, 163
hypoglycemia, 163
lactogenesis II delay, 162
weight loss, 162, 163
supplementation, 161
tapering, 172
temporary, 162
twins, 177
volume, 164
supplemental nursing systems
(SNS), 85, 168–172
advantages, 169–170
breast milk removal, 169
interruption need, 169

skin-to-skin contact, 169
triple feeding method, 169–170
disadvantages, 170
no. 5 French feeding tube, 168
use of, 170–172
nipple shields, 170
plunger, 171
supplements, 161, 189
surfactant production, 42–43, 45
alveolar collapse, 42
breastfeeding, 42
lung development, 43
phospholipids, 42
sustained suckling patterns, 125
synapsed afferent axonal terminals, 19
synaptic firings, effect on breastfeeding, 22
synaptogenesis, 19
synthetic oxytocin. *See* pitocin
syringes, 168
as feeding medium, 166
systemic lupus erythematosus (SLE), 13
premature rupture of membranes, 13

tachynpea, 29, 44
causes, 44
burping, 44
glucose conversion, 44
hyperthermia, 44
hypotonia, 44
sepsis, 44
trachea distortion, 44
tandem feeding, 176
tapering, supplemental feeding and, 172
temperature instability, 51
bilirubin and, 37
temperature stability. *See* thermoregulation
Ten Steps to Successful Breastfeeding, 81,82, 84

theca lutein cysts, 59
thermoregulation, 25–28, 96
adult, 26
brown fat, 26
hyperthermia, 25
hypoglycemia, 25
hypothermia, 25
subcutaneous fat, 26–27
thyroid, 57
disease, 13
galactopoietic response, 57
prolactin, 57
tight frenulum, 178–179
breastfeeding success, 179
significance of, 178–179
treatment of, 179
Tommee Tippee nipple shields, 126–127
tongue tie, 178–179
tongue, peristaltic action of, 124
total serum bilirubin (TSB), 37
hyperbilirubinemia, 37
lactogenesis II, 37
trachea, distortion of, 44
transcutaneous bilirubin, 89
transient tachynpea of the newborn (TTN), 42, 43, 46
cesarean delivery, 43
fetal lung fluid, 43
tremors, 29
triglyceride oxidation, 26, 27
oxygen consumption, 27
triglycerides, 26, 71
triple feeding method, 169–170
triplets, 62
sharing breast, 176
supplemental feeding of, 177
TSB. *See* total serum bilirubin
TTN. *See* transient tachypnea of the newborn
twins, 62, 175–178
breast sharing, 176
supplemental feeding, 177

ultrathin nipple shields, 121–124
  application of, 128–132
    sizing, 128–129
  breastfeeding termination, 124
  cautionary notes, 134–135
  choking prevention, 125
  effectiveness of, 121–123
  latching, 132–134
  milk flow, 125
  prolactin levels, 124
  sustained suckling patterns, 125
  termination of, 133–134
  types, 126–128
    Avent, 126
    Ameda, 126
    contact, 127–128
    Dr. Brown's, 127
    full-term infants vs. late
      preterm, 126
    Medela, 126
    regular, 127–128
    Tommee Tippee, 126–127
  use of, 129–132
  value of, 124
  weaning, 134
unbound lipid-soluble bilirubin, 38
unconjugated bilirubin, 34
  levels, 37, 38
underdeveloped breasts, 54
UNICEF. *See* United Nations
    Children's Fund.
United Nations Children's Fund
    (UNICEF), 81
unstable respiratory function, 45
  breastfeeding, 45
    mother–baby separation, 45–46
  metabolic demand, 46
    nothing by mouth, 46
    transient tachynpea of the
      newborn, 46

upper airway dilatory muscle tone,
    decreased, 44
uridine diphosate glucuronyl
    transferase, 33

vacuum pressure, 145, 147, 148
vacuum pump, 146
  pressure, 147–148
vasodilators, 12
ventilator-treated respiratory
    distress, 42
volumes, feeding supplements, 164

wake cycles, 115
water-soluble bilirubin, 34
weak suck, 53
weaning, 134
weight loss, 89, 162, 163
white blood cells, 90
  polymorphonucleocytes, 90
white matter
  maturation of, 19
  myelinated axons, 19
  myelination of the spinal cord, 19
WHO. *See* World Health
    Organization
WIC. *See* Women, Infants, and
    Children nutrition program
Women, Infants, and Children (WIC)
    nutrition program, 66
World Health Organization (WHO),
    14, 81, 82
  worldwide preterm statistics, 4

yeast infections, 51